Authorized to Heal

Gender, Class,

and the

Transformation

of Medicine

in Appalachia,

1880–1930

Sandra Lee Barney

The University of North Carolina Press

Chapel Hill and London

© 2000 The University of North Carolina Press

All rights reserved

Manufactured in the United States of America

Designed by April Leidig-Higgins

Set in Monotype Joanna

by Keystone Typesetting, Inc.

The paper in this book meets the guidelines for permanence and durability of the Committee on Production Guidelines for Book Longevity of the Council on Library Resources.

Library of Congress Cataloging-in-Publication Data
Barney, Sandra. Authorized to heal : gender, class, and the transformation of medicine in Appalachia, 1880–1930 / Sandra Lee Barney.
p. cm. Includes bibliographical references and index.
ISBN 0-8078-2522-0 (cloth : alk. paper).
ISBN 0-8078-4834-4 (paper : alk. paper)
1. Women in medicine—Appalachian Region—History.
2. Medicine—Appalachian Region—History. I. Title.
R692.B67 2000   362.1'0974—dc21   99-30433 CIP

04 03 02 01 00   5 4 3 2 1

CONTENTS

ILLUSTRATIONS

TABLES

ACKNOWLEDGMENTS   .

Like everyone who writes a book, I have incurred debts that can never be repaid. Although it is impossible to name all of the people who helped me with this project, I offer a public "thank you" as a small symbol of my gratitude.

Whatever skills I possess as a writer or scholar have their origins in my undergraduate experience at Auburn University. When I was straight off the farm, Joseph Kicklighter, Allen Cronenberg, Hines Hall, Wayne Flynt, Ruth Crocker, and especially Donna Bohanan modeled dedicated scholarship and good teaching for me. I only hope I can show my students the same generosity these professors extended to me and inspire in them the same curiosity that was instilled in me. Roger Williams and Robert Righter at the University of Wyoming taught me a great deal about writing and showed me just how much I had to learn to become a real historian.

Ronald L. Lewis was my dissertation adviser at West Virginia University, and I count having the opportunity to work with him the greatest fortune of my academic career. His intellect and dedication are surpassed only by his concern for his students and for the discipline of Appalachian studies. The other members of my dissertation committee, Elizabeth Fones-Wolf, Gregory Good, Mary Lou Lustig, and Sally Ward Maggard, all offered thoughtful insights and gentle direction.

Without the guidance of a number of archivists, this work would never have been completed. I am especially grateful to reference librarian Todd Yeager at West Virginia University; Christelle Venham and the staff at the West Virginia and Regional History Collection at West Virginia University; Cindy Swanson at the General Federation of Women's Clubs Women's History and Resource Center in Washington, D.C.; Aloha South at the National Archives and Records Administration; Gerald Roberts, Sidney Saylor Farr, and Shannon Wilson at the Southern Appalachian Archives at Berea College; and the staff of the Kentucky State Department of Libraries and Archives. Jodi Koste at the Medical College of Virginia Archives and Mary Kay

Becker at the Kornhauser Health Sciences Library at the University of Louisville offered me thoughtful research direction as well as archival help. Both came through at critical moments and went well beyond the call of duty. Nancy Hill of the West Virginia State Medical Association and Ola Powers of the Virginia State Board of Medicine allowed me access to their records and were always kind hostesses during my visits. I appreciate the professional services these people provided, but I am especially thankful for their interest in my project.

During the preparation of the manuscript, several people were kind enough to read portions of it. Barbara Ellen Smith, Sally Ward Maggard, Hallie Chillag, Shaunna Scott, Anne-Marie Turnage, and Janet Irons all offered thoughtful comments. Richard Couto read the initial draft and, along with an anonymous second reader, made insightful suggestions.

I have found that some of the greatest revelations about this project have evolved from conversations with friends and colleagues. My graduate school companions, Jim Cook, Jerra Jenrette, Paul Rakes, and Deborah Weiner, challenged me both inside and outside the classroom. John Hennen still serves as my model of a dedicated scholar-activist. Since completing my degree, I have been fortunate enough to meet a number of individuals who have pushed me to think about this project in more sophisticated ways. Janet Irons and Nan Elizabeth Woodruff, southern historians who share my northern exile, have challenged and supported me on many levels. Jennifer Gunn, Elizabeth Toon, and Lynne Snyder have encouraged me to recognize the importance of the scholarship on the history of medicine to this work.

My friend Nan Woodruff likes to say that she became an academic so she could be around interesting people. I agree and have been blessed by the support of many interesting people who assisted with this project in one way or another. Mary Lou Lustig, Sally Ward Maggard, Rachel Tompkins, and Hallie Chillag have been more than colleagues or advisers; they have been dear friends, and nothing in my life, this book included, would ever be accomplished without their assistance. Jill Pearce Jordan, college roommate and sometimes financial savior, does not understand just what academics do, but she is glad I found gainful employment.

Sian Hunter, my acquisitions editor at the University of North Carolina Press, has been a wonderful guide throughout the publication process. More important, she has become a friend. I appreciate the work of the entire staff of UNC Press. Any errors or omissions that may remain, however, are my own.

Finally, my greatest thanks go to Anne-Marie Turnage, who has lived with this project as long as I have. My best ideas are probably hers, and whatever incorrect presumptions persist have been retained over her objections. Without her intellectual insight, good sense, and patience, I would never have completed this manuscript. Now it's her turn to retreat to the attic to write.

AUTHORIZED TO HEAL

In 1932, the West Virginia Federation of Women's Clubs announced its intention to help reform the state's tuberculosis sanatoriums, "thereby accepting the findings of Medical Science."[1] The middle-class wives and mothers of lawyers, doctors, shop owners, newspaper editors, and coal operators who dominated this voluntary association were inspired by the promises of scientific medicine and vowed to carry the "True Story of Medicine" to their communities and to champion its adoption by Appalachian people of all social classes and geographical circumstances.[2]

In proclaiming their loyalty to the ideals of scientific medicine, these women echoed the pronouncements of doctors, public health officials, nurses, and other health promoters who had campaigned for the fundamental reconstruction of health care in Appalachia during the period from 1880 to 1930. These constituencies sometimes articulated conflicting ambitions but often united in public insistence that improvements in medicine could deliver to rural Appalachian people benefits that previously had been denied them by isolation, poverty, and the absence of trained physicians.[3] This coalition eventually fractured along complicated gender, class, and professional lines, but before it collapsed, its members joined the native Appalachians and recently arrived industrial workers who populated the region to re-create medical care in Appalachia. In the process, mountain residents developed presumptions about the efficacy and delivery of medicine that placed their region squarely within the evolving American mainstream.[4]

By offering a new comprehension of the role of various female constituencies in the campaign to elevate scientific medicine in Appalachia during the era of industrial transformation, this work begins to fill a void in Appalachian history. I attempt to illuminate the class and professional tensions that divided women, as well as to consider the common ground that connected them to one another and to the male physicians who profited from their voluntary activity. Building on the work of Mary Anglin, Jane Becker, Sally Ward

Maggard, Barbara Ellen Smith, and Karen Tice, I evaluate the tactics and actions of various female reform constituencies and explore how gender, class, professional status, kinship, and friendship shaped their reform goals and strategies. I also demonstrate how class identity defined relationships among women who were targeted to receive benevolence, female caregivers whose skills and economic activities were devalued and displaced by reformers, and women who used benevolence work to facilitate their entry into the middle class.[5] Ultimately, I intend to illustrate that class and professional status joined with gender to define women's actions. I also argue that the decline of a reform agenda among middle-class women and the culmination of medical professionalization eventually undermined reform efforts in the 1920s, an argument in keeping with recent scholarship on maternalist policies in general.[6]

This examination of the transformation of medicine in Appalachia from 1880 to 1930 is situated at the nexus of three historiographical literatures. To describe the status of medical care in the nineteenth century and the dramatic changes that reshaped it, I have drawn heavily from literature on the history of medicine, especially from scholars who have examined the importance of public health and the decline of midwifery. Their work defines the first two chapters of this book. The remaining chapters are influenced by the rich history of gender and maternalism produced in the late 1980s and 1990s. The book responds most specifically to Theda Skocpol's call for regional and local studies of women's activism outside the nation's urban centers during the first decades of the twentieth century.[7] Overarching both of these literatures is the increasingly sophisticated historiography of Appalachian studies. It is in that literature that this work is most firmly grounded.

By examining the professionalization of male medical practitioners, the gendered nature of the campaign to promote their hegemony, and their displacement of community healers, especially female midwives, I hope to illuminate some of the tensions that evolved within Appalachian society as the region was fundamentally reshaped during the era of industrial development. Unlike most analyses of Appalachian history during these decades, however, this work does not focus on traditional sites of conflict, although many of the male subjects of this study were employed by coal or timber operations and the political manipulations of the day undoubtedly impacted the displacement of traditional healers. My goal instead is to broaden our understanding of the transformation of Appalachia to include a recognition of the effects of change on relations between professionals and those who never secured professional legitimacy and on interaction between the sexes as well as among women of different class and professional standings.[8]

The arrival of railroads, the development of commercial timber exploitation, and the enormous growth of the coal industry unquestionably defined the transformation of medical care in the Central Appalachian counties of eastern Kentucky, southern West Virginia, and southwestern Virginia during this era.[9] As scholars such as John Gaventa and Ronald Eller have demonstrated, the introduction of railroads linking Appalachian resources to external markets at the end of the nineteenth century had both intensive and extensive consequences for the region.[10] Although the scholarship of Wilma Dunaway, Kenneth Noe, Paul Salstrom, and John Inscoe has revealed that the Appalachian economy was linked to regional, national, and global markets before the industrial transformation occurred, Ronald L. Lewis has convincingly argued that such linkages were not comprehensive enough to fundamentally remake life in the mountains in the way that large-scale coal and timber extraction did.[11]

Mary Beth Pudup, Dwight Billings, and Altina Waller point out in their introduction to *Appalachia in the Making*, however, that the commercial activity documented by Dunaway, Noe, and others was substantial enough to create a class of local elites and early entrepreneurs who facilitated the introduction of outside capital into Appalachia. Their argument builds on Pudup's earlier work on class in preindustrial Appalachia, which held that time of settlement, possession of land, occupational status, and family prestige combined to confer class status on Appalachian residents.[12] It was this established sector of the Appalachian population, often ignored or dismissed by many historians as collaborators who fostered the exploitation of the region, that produced many of the early physicians who served mountain residents.[13]

As medical historians have demonstrated, most nineteenth-century physicians derived their professional legitimacy from their affiliation with their school of practice and their social standing. "The physician's effectiveness as a healer," medical historian John Harley Warner has written, "was thought to depend as much on who he was as what he knew."[14] Appalachian physicians were no different. Like their rural colleagues elsewhere, many early practitioners received their training through private apprenticeship with preceptors and only took brief medical courses, if they matriculated in formal medical schools at all.[15]

Equipped with little formal training, nineteenth-century Appalachian physicians acquired their social standing and economic stability through a complicated mix of professional accomplishment, family position, agricultural activity, and ancillary economic ventures.[16] Physicians whose families owned agricultural land or had an interest in early commercial endeavors such as salt extraction or timbering depended on their medical practices to further protect their economic position.[17] Those whose families were less privileged or who attempted to rely on their private practices alone often found themselves in difficult circumstances; some were unable to meet their debts, and others abandoned the medical profession and pursued more financially rewarding endeavors, picking up or discarding the mantle of medical practitioner as needed or desired.[18]

Before the arrival of railroads, Appalachian physicians, disadvantaged in their professional development by their isolation and the relative poverty of most of their potential patients, struggled for occupational security.[19] The dramatic rise in population created by the coal boom in the last decades of the nineteenth century offered doctors rich new fields in which to pursue their developing profession, and workers' employment in the cash economy eliminated many of the prohibitive costs that previously had deterred Appalachian people from seeking care from regularly trained physicians.[20] Unlike the generally stable communities that had existed before the Civil War, however, these new settlements were inhabited by foreign immigrants, African Americans who had fled Jim Crow for the relative freedom of the Upper South, and mountaineers negotiating a place for themselves in the developing industrial order.[21] The congregation of large numbers of potential patients in company towns and growing county seats created new economic opportunities for physicians, but ambitious doctors, especially those who moved into the region from outside, had to concoct innovative ways to claim legitimacy for themselves in towns and coal camps often filled with strangers.[22]

Warner has demonstrated that the medical profession was undergoing an epistemological shift in the last decades of the nineteenth century as new scientific discoveries challenged earlier presumptions about diagnosis and therapy. By the beginning of the coal boom, many elite physicians, especially those near traditional centers of medical education, had dismissed their heroic therapies and their reliance on specificity and were eagerly awaiting new scientific advances that would augment their therapeutic arsenal.[23] As popular support for the claims of scientific medicine grew around the turn of the century, many younger doctors and medical students quickly embraced the promise of science, even though they had not yet secured real knowledge of its applications.

Charlotte Borst has argued that the "rhetoric of the scientifically educated physician far outran the reality."[24] Her claim is certainly supported by an evaluation of the medical education received by many Appalachian physicians before the turn of the century. The dramatic changes debated among elite medical practitioners had few real consequences for rural physicians far removed from the centers of medical education like those who practiced in Appalachia.

Historians have demonstrated that reformers at elite institutions led successful campaigns to create new, more rigorous medical curricula firmly grounded in the German clinical tradition.[25] Students at the Medical College of Virginia, the University of Louisville, and the College of Physicians and Surgeons in Baltimore, the three institutions that educated the majority of Appalachian doctors during the years under scrutiny, however, experienced a very different medical education. Their training was defined by the didactic tradition, and many of their professors were still guided by the clinical perspective associated with French medical practice that had dominated American medical education in the middle decades of the nineteenth century.[26] Such instructors were slow to embrace reform, and their curricula bore little resemblance to the scientifically oriented course of study that was becoming the ideal in American medical education by the 1890s.[27]

Although the education most Appalachian physicians received before 1910 had little in common with the reformed curricula of elite schools that historians have typically highlighted, it did provide ambitious doctors with an important tool for negotiating their way into the developing middle class. Many Appalachian doctors had little training in the laboratory sciences, but they still proclaimed themselves advocates of science and pitched their tents under its banner as they battled to build a unique identity as professional physicians and to achieve status as members of the middle class.

Before the investment of large amounts of capital in the development of the coal industry, Pudup argues, few markets for "centralized, specialized economic activities in Appalachia" existed.[28] Such circumstances, Paul Starr asserts, deterred the professional development of medical practitioners and forced physicians to seek income from outside sources.[29] The advent of timber and coal extraction and the connection of the region to the rest of the nation through railroads fundamentally altered those conditions. The acquisition of a medical degree helped doctors who were native to the region and whose families possessed significant social and economic capital to elevate or protect their status as their communities were changed by the arrival of new industrial workers and outside investors.[30]

Non-native physicians who moved to Appalachia after completing medical school were even more dependent on the legitimacy they claimed as scientific medical practitioners than were local doctors. Without familial and community ties in the region, the young physicians who came to Appalachia to work on railroads or in coal camps or to establish independent private practices in bustling new towns had only their medical credentials to legitimize their activities. For these young men, possession of scientific medical knowledge was the most important, and often the only, asset they had to rely on as they sought to make a living.[31]

Physicians struggled to establish themselves on two fronts in these growing communities. They sought camaraderie with and entrée into the region's developing professional and middle class. Many physicians were accepted by the mine operators, engineers, lawyers, newspaper editors, and merchants who made up the region's growing middle class as fellow professionals who shared the same class and economic interests.[32] Doctors worked to secure their fortunes by fostering these alliances, forging an identity distinct from the working-class allegiance being formed in the coal camps.[33]

Physicians labored to elevate themselves above the working and farming classes and to claim the title "professional," but to do so, they needed recognition from these same populations. With the intrusion of industrial capitalism into Central Appalachia at the end of the nineteenth century, the workers and residents of the mountains discovered that the self-sufficient existence they had shared with many other rural Americans was coming to an end and that they had to look to experts to provide services they had previously supplied for themselves.[34] Desiring the advantages promised by scientific medicine, Appalachian people constituted a significant potential market for ambitious doctors.

In *The Culture of Professionalism*, Burton Bledstein argues that professionalization entails the transformation of occupational practice from "distributing a commodity to offering a service based on acquired skill."[35] To make that shift, Eliot Friedson claims, practitioners of an occupation must exhibit expert knowledge, possess a recognized system of credentialing, and have the autonomy to define the standards as well as the knowledge of the discipline.[36] At the beginning of the coal boom, Appalachian physicians possessed the desire to upgrade their occupation but little else. To make the shift to full professional status, physicians had to consolidate and agree on an accepted body of knowledge, construct institutions and agencies to formulate and evaluate credentials, and secure recognition as the only agents who could authoritatively speak to or about their field.

Although the scientific advances that reshaped medical education influenced developments within medicine, they did not always immediately translate into observable benefits for laypeople. Charles Rosenberg argues that "the faith of many progressives in science was a real one," but "the appeal of science . . . was largely limited to the educated, the elite and the articulate. Science did not appeal with equal cogency to . . . [the] provincial."[37] As physicians struggled to reconcile new scientific knowledge with established traditions of practice, the dissension within their ranks discouraged potential clients who were already burdened by the lack of disposable cash for medical services and little knowledge of the medical system.

To Appalachian farmers who were still at least partially entangled in subsistence farming, rumors about the benefit of scientific medicine were attractive, but they paled in comparison with the enormous difficulties a family faced when trying to secure cash with which to pay a doctor.[38] Confronted by what Starr has called the "real cost of medicine," many farmers continued to reject professional physicians in favor of local healers.[39]

Many residents of mountain communities did not encounter a formally trained professional doctor until the coal boom[40] Assistance at childbirth was a traditional method for a physician to begin building a relationship with a family, but unlike the southern women Sally McMillen investigated and the northern families Sylvia Hoffert studied, relatively few Appalachian women relied on physicians to deliver their babies before the end of the nineteenth century. Instead, as Borst's study of midwifery in Wisconsin has demonstrated, most still patronized midwives and had not yet come to rely on the male accoucheur.[41]

Appalachian residents who were disinclined to abandon traditional health care providers possessed what Judith Walzer Leavitt has called a "rival worldview."[42] Just as Typhoid Mary Mallon rejected physicians' claims that she was ill even though she felt well, some Appalachian people distrusted the unknowable, mysterious agents that doctors increasingly blamed for illness. Unprepared by education or training to comprehend the principles on which new remedies were based, resistant mountaineers took refuge in traditional cures. Some rejected all treatments and fell back on a religious fatalism that fostered an overly simplistic stereotype of Appalachians as opponents of progress.[43]

Such a stereotype fails to recognize that, like many laypeople in the United States, Appalachian residents were attempting to interpret the sometimes conflicting information they received from practitioners.[44] Sectarians such as homeopaths and eclectics competed with regular physicians in the nineteenth century, but differences of opinion about diagnosis and therapy also divided regular physicians. When younger doctors who were better versed in scientific medicine arrived in the mountains, they found themselves in conflict with older doctors who did not share their commitment to the germ theory of disease. As the two forces debated the validity of vaccinations and quarantines, puzzled onlookers pondered the meaning and authority of medical care.[45]

Frustrated by the recalcitrance of their predecessors, younger Appalachian physicians initiated efforts to establish a professional identity. A doctor's medical diploma, "an instrument of ambition and a vehicle to status in the occupational world," served as a symbol of the expert knowledge doctors possessed.[46] Younger physicians also organized local chapters of the American Medical Association to foster camaraderie among educated regular doctors. Professionally ambitious doctors agitated for the establishment and enforcement of formal licensing requirements that acknowledged the importance of medical education and subjugated competing medical philosophies to the absolutes of scientific medicine.

These efforts improved the professional standing of Appalachian physicians, but they failed to secure the autonomy that Friedson identifies as the last step in professional development. For physicians to achieve that goal, Appalachian people had to accept, "by choice or sufferance, the professional definition of both [their] needs and the means to satisfy them."[47]

The drive by physicians to displace lay midwives clearly illustrates doctors' determination to impose their "professional definition" on the Appalachian psyche. As a number of historians have documented, midwives were the standard of care throughout much of the United States until the first decades of the twentieth century.[48] For many Appalachian physicians, the midwife "carried the stigma of the pre-modern culture."[49] If doctors were to be seen as the only legitimate childbirth attendants, they had to encourage mothers, and by extension their families, to reject midwifery and embrace modern, scientific medicine. But to accomplish such a drastic cultural change, physicians had to look outside their professional ranks for volunteers from their social and economic class to assist them in reshaping expectations about health and healing.[50]

Driven by maternalist goals, middle-class reformers and their confederates in the settlement movement welcomed the opportunity to promote the advantages of scientific medicine to those less fortunate than themselves.[51] Physicians profited from women's reform work, and female associations benefited from their affiliation with doctors. Kathryn Kish Sklar has convincingly argued that reform-minded "women needed access to the institutional power and positions of public authority that men held and men needed the grassroots support that women could mobilize."[52] Middle-class female reformers furthered the professional aims of doctors while pursuing their own plans to remake working-class and immigrant women into their image of Anglo-Saxon "good mothers."[53]

The women involved in the crusade to improve medical conditions in the mountains can be divided into three categories: members of the General Federation of Women's Clubs, a group drawn primarily from the growing middle class that developed as a consequence of industrial expansion; educated, and often wealthy, women who led the early settlement school movement; and public health nurses and female physicians who saw the expansion of medical care as a possible source of professional opportunity. Each of these groups possessed a unique vision of how new developments in medical science should be delivered and of who should control their application, but cooperation among them was frequent and critical to the success of many projects. As Skocpol has demonstrated in her studies of women reformers at the national level, middle-class Appalachian clubwomen provided grassroots support for programs administered by well-educated members of the regional settlement movement elite.[54]

For middle-class clubwomen and the wives of physicians who

joined both independent women's groups and subordinate auxiliaries of medical associations, clubs allowed newcomers who had followed their husbands or fathers to the coalfields to continue traditions of benevolence they had learned elsewhere. Local women whose male relatives profited from land sales or acquisition of gainful positions with railroads, coal mines, or timber operations joined these newcomers in their benevolence work, creating a new coalition that fostered their "identity as local boosters."[55]

Appalachian clubwomen initiated a plethora of programs to educate working-class mothers about prenatal and infant care and to provide preventive screenings and examinations for children during the first decades of the twentieth century. Focusing much of their attention on improving maternal health, these reformers promoted an agenda defined by the belief that good mothering included an appropriate amount of deference to scientific authority.[56] Legitimizing their efforts by presenting them as extensions of their duties as wives and mothers, middle-class women reduced both the "conflict between public and home responsibilities" and the probability that they would be charged with "neglecting home duties."[57] These women's promotion of scientific medicine could be portrayed and interpreted as a campaign to extend benefits they had already secured for themselves to those they perceived to be less fortunate than themselves.[58] By joining with other American women in municipal housekeeping and community amelioration activities, Appalachian clubwomen assured themselves that they, like women volunteers in the nineteenth century, were "carrying out the responsibilities appropriate to wives and daughters of community leaders," a status they sought in the rapidly expanding towns and villages of Central Appalachia.[59]

If middle-class women used their benevolence work to elevate their status while helping the community, the educated women who initiated secular settlement work in the hills of Appalachia sought other gratification.[60] These women, peripheral members of the reform elite described by Robyn Muncy, sought to apply the social service principles developed at urban settlements in Appalachian communities.[61] Like Jane Addams, Ellen Gates Starr, and Vida Scudder, women such as May Stone, Katherine Pettit, and Lucy Furman who founded and guided mountain settlement work at the beginning of the twentieth century constructed complicated identities within the multilayered contexts in which they lived and worked.[62]

Born and educated outside Appalachia, these independent women attempted to create new opportunities for fulfilling work at the same time that they attacked the poverty and cultural deprivation they identified in the mountains.[63] Appalachian settlement workers, like settlement workers in urban areas, used their education and their social and economic standing to claim legitimacy as agents of cultural change.[64] By allying themselves with physicians, they could bring critically needed services to Appalachia's most remote communities while fostering ties with potential allies who could provide public, and perhaps financial, support for their projects.

As Karen Tice has argued, settlement workers functioned in a number of contexts and assumed complicated identities that reflected their experiences both inside and outside mountain communities.[65] At the Pine Mountain, Hindman, and Caney Creek Settlement Schools, for example, public health nurses were employed to provide professional medical services such as vaccinations and emergency first aid, but they were also expected to participate in educational and cultural work.[66]

Mary Breckinridge, who founded the Frontier Nursing Service, possessed wealth and prestige equal or superior to the wealth and prestige of the women who founded the mountain settlement schools. Her legitimacy, however, came from her professional training as a nurse-midwife as well as from her family name and wealth.[67] Her registration as a nurse-midwife, entered on a physician's license form revised in ink, stands as a telling reminder of her determination to be recognized for her professional credentials even though Leslie County, Kentucky, had no established procedure for acknowledging her achievements.[68]

Acquisition of professional status for Breckinridge and other nurse-midwives of the Frontier Nursing Service was part of a larger plan to further the work of that organization in the mountains. For many nurses and female physicians, however, professional recognition also meant economic stability. Like male doctors, these women sought to acquire new status in the community based on their possession of specialized knowledge and their completion of formal training. Many male physicians secured work in industrial contexts, but female public health nurses and doctors often sought to acquire professional standing through employment in state and private public health agencies, forging a uniquely feminine definition of professionalism, as Muncy has documented.[69]

Advocacy of public health projects, like all professional campaigns by medical providers in this era, was altruistic as well as self-serving. Public health programs, especially gender-specific programs such as maternal and infant health work, provided critical services to poor and isolated Appalachian women; at the same time, their altruism demonstrated the special abilities of public health nurses, who often conducted the work with minimal supervision. At the administrative level, the female physicians who ran such programs gained significant recognition and professional affirmation.[70]

The public health and educational programs administered by women reformers helped male physicians achieve the hegemony they had strived to acquire since the late nineteenth century. Ironically, male physicians sought to control programs administered by women to serve women because such efforts were so successful. Through the medical services they provided to working-class families and isolated mountain homes, women health activists carried a message of dependency on and deference to the professional physician. As Sheila Rothman argued in 1978 and Theda Skocpol and Richard Meckel have recently reminded us, the termination of programs targeted at and administered by women in the 1920s signaled both a rejection of publicly funded medical care and a denial of the concept that women's maternalist qualifications authorized them to speak on health matters.[71]

Having cooperated with women reformers to acquire the autonomy they needed to solidify their professional status, male physicians used their recently secured autonomy to silence their former allies. By the 1930s, women's clubs pursued relatively few health initiatives, and physicians increasingly relied on their dependent women's auxiliaries to promote a new health care message that focused on furthering the physician's professional status.

But women were not passive victims driven from work they loved by tyrannical physicians. Sklar has written that women's reform efforts before 1920 were "sustained by beliefs associated with women's political culture. When those beliefs were washed away by a sea change in values affecting gender identity and gender relations during the 1920s, so too was much of the power of women's political culture."[72]

By the end of the 1920s, physicians and their class allies in Appalachia reigned over a maturing social system that they had been slowly constructing since commercial timber and coal extraction was initiated in the late nineteenth century. With miners and their families firmly established in coal camps and the labor unrest of the post–World War I era suppressed, middle-class Appalachians were free to enjoy the fruits of their labors by joining other Americans in an orgy of consumption and conservatism.[73]

Through their assistance in the promotion of a new medical model in Appalachia, women reformers were aiding in the birth of the middle-class culture that came to dominate Appalachia during the first decades of the twentieth century. In *The Americanization of West Virginia*, John Hennen has demonstrated that women volunteers were key actors in the campaign by industrial elites to produce a quiescent working class. I argue that the promotion of reliance on the male-dominated, professional medical model was part and parcel of the same campaign. By encouraging dependence on a bureaucratized medical system controlled by a relatively small faction of the population, women reformers furthered the industrial elite's ambitions at the same time that they helped purchase a prosperous position for themselves and their families as members of the Appalachian middle class.[74]

To trace the evolution of medicine in the mountains and the role of women volunteers in advancing the new medical model, I have followed a chronological format that fortunately fits into a thematic one as well. Chapter 1 describes the state of medicine before industrialization and addresses the importance of expansion based on extractive industries to the region and to physicians. Chapter 2 introduces the campaign by physicians to construct a professional identity through reliance on their improving medical education, the creation of private medical societies, and their alliance with the state to enact licensing requirements that excluded other schools of medical practice as well as lay healers. Unable to bring about the broad cultural changes that would encourage mountain residents to rely on trained physicians alone, doctors began to reach out to their class allies. The growth and development of the women's clubs and settlement schools that were so important to physicians' efforts are described in chapter 3. The educational and preventive programs initiated by female reformers and the complicated negotiations with physicians, nurses, and targeted recipients they had to engage in to achieve their goals are addressed in chapter 4. The final chapter describes physicians' growing antagonism toward public health initiatives and the erosion of laywomen's support for health advocacy in the 1920s. The conclusion discusses the formalization of physicians' power in the decades after the 1920s and considers the consequences of their success for Appalachian residents, focusing on the failure of gender-based alliances to protect women's interests from the medical monopoly.

CHAPTER ONE

Bringing

Modern

Medicine to

the Mountains

In the opening scene of Harriet Arnow's Appalachian classic, *The Dollmaker*, the heroine Gertie Nevels saves her young son's life by performing a rude tracheotomy on him with a pocketknife. This desperate act shocks the soldiers Gertie has compelled to help her transport the child to the nearest physician many miles from her country home. Having internalized modern ideas about medical care, the soldiers presume that only a physician can perform such an operation. Gertie shares the soldiers' belief that a professional practitioner is the preferred medical provider, but she retains the skills necessary to respond to a crisis independently.[1]

Appalachian people maintained these skills in the twentieth century because, like many rural people across the United States, they had little contact with well-educated, professional physicians before the end of the nineteenth century.[2] Too scattered in small communities and on mountain farms to attract significant numbers of practitioners, mountaineers turned to the few physicians, whether trained or uneducated, who lived in their counties or districts for treatment of illnesses or injuries that seemed beyond the abilities of domestic or lay healers.[3]

The physicians who practiced in Appalachia before the arrival of industrial capitalism bore a striking resemblance to doctors who practiced in other rural areas of the United States during this era. The quality of their formal educations varied widely, they were defined by their allegiance to a unique philosophy of practice rather than by their possession of significant medical knowledge, and many depended on family connections or alternative economic and social activities for financial security. Few relied on their medical practices alone for support, and when they did attempt to define themselves exclusively as medical practitioners, they often faced significant economic difficulties.[4]

In some part, their economic vulnerability was rooted in the impotence of their treatments. Because of the decline in reliance on harsh heroic methods used in the West since ancient times and the relatively slow pace of medical innovation before the Civil War, mountain doctors had few efficacious weapons, or even visibly active therapies, with which to treat illness.[5] Deterred by the cost of medical care and uninterested in the few advantages it seemed to offer, rural mountaineers continued to turn to traditional caregivers, seeking professional medical help only when all other treatments failed.

The coexistence of these two medical traditions was fundamentally challenged in the last two decades of the nineteenth century by a combination of developments that reflected the maturing of science and technology in the United States. As the growth and eventual dominance of industrial capitalism reshaped American society, Appalachia finally became fully invested in the national market. Identified as a critical source of fuel to feed the burgeoning manufacturing sector, Appalachia was reconstructed by the acquisition and exploitation of coal and, to a lesser extent, timber.[6] The environmental, social, economic, and political repercussions of the new position Appalachia was assigned in the national economy were enormous, and they re-created life in the region, providing new markets and population centers for aspiring professionals.

At the same time, medicine was undergoing a fundamental transformation in which reliance on empiricism was replaced by a new regard for scientific principles, an alteration that legitimized new therapeutic presumptions as well as elevating the status of the medical profession.[7] Doctors also welcomed these developments because they justified physicians' efforts to secure economic stability by demonstrating that educated physicians did indeed possess unique skills worthy of financial compensation.

The scientific advances of the 1880s and 1890s began to bolster younger, better educated physicians' claims that they possessed special knowledge of what Paul Starr has called the "legitimate complexity" of medicine. These advances, however, were slow to trickle down to schools such as the University of Louisville, the Medical

Bringing Modern Medicine to the Mountains

College of Virginia, and the College of Physicians and Surgeons in Baltimore, which trained about half of the Appalachian physicians who practiced before 1925.[8] Although graduates of these schools at the end of the century had few real scientific credentials, ambitious young physicians, seeing the economic opportunities available in the coalfields, proclaimed themselves apostles of science and set out to find economic security and professional standing there.

These young physicians, coming from both native families and outside the region, were critical actors in the creation of a new Appalachian middle class. Determined to construct secure professional identities based on their possession of specialized scientific knowledge, they rejected the methods of older Appalachian physicians and sought to replace them as bearers of the medical standard and recipients of available health care expenditures. To develop their practices and expand their clientele, many gained employment with railroads, the earliest overt symbol of industrial intrusion, or later acquired positions with coal or timber companies. These assignments provided them with paychecks, opportunities to invest in industrial development, close contact with other members of the nascent middle class, and the security to pursue the advancement of membership in professional organizations and alliances with government that would foster their authority as sole claimants to the title "doctor."

Before the introduction of large-scale resource extraction at the end of the nineteenth century, few physicians practiced in the mountains. The scarcity of professional medical care before industrialization was a direct result of the low population of Central Appalachia at that time. Not surprisingly, small communities could not attract the gradually improving medical care available in cities and prosperous commercial farming centers. The 5,371 inhabitants of Harlan County, Kentucky, for example, were served by only one doctor in 1860. Like the other thirty-one men in the county who identified themselves as professionals in the manuscript census that year, Harlan County's physician did not rely solely on his trade but also engaged in farming.[9] The situation in Harlan was not unusual. In the years during and immediately after the Civil War, no more than one formally recognized physician at a time resided in Perry County, Kentucky. According to the 1880 census, that number had doubled by the end of the 1870s. Nearby Floyd County, Kentucky, with its commercial center at Prestonsburg, enjoyed a relative abundance of medical care. Four physicians practiced there on the eve of the Civil War; the number dropped to two by 1870 but mushroomed to eight by 1880.[10]

Population size alone does not fully explain the low number of formally trained physicians practicing in Central Appalachia. As author Wilma Dunaway has demonstrated, by the eve of the Civil War, the majority of Appalachian people were landless and without significant wealth.[11] Unlike affluent commercial farmers and members of the growing urban middle class and elite, residents of most nineteenth-century mountain communities were unable to offer the sort of financial incentives that would attract significant numbers of well-educated physicians.

According to Dunaway, Appalachia was one of the poorest regions of the United States just before the Civil War. Mountain citizens possessed only half of the wealth enjoyed by average Americans and lagged behind other southerners in income and property as well. Already vulnerable to shifting regional, national, and world markets, Appalachian residents occupied a precarious position that provided little disposable currency for the purchase of professional goods and services.[12]

The lack of occupational specialization noted in the nineteenth-century censuses of the region reveals the inability of mountain residents to pay for medical care or other professional services. In 1860, the percentages of residents pursuing nonfarming occupations in Floyd, Harlan, and Perry Counties in Kentucky were 1 percent, .5 percent, and .4 percent, respectively. The nonfarming category included shoemakers, tavernkeepers, clerks, mechanics, and saddlers as well as more commonly identified professionals such as lawyers, teachers, businesspeople, and doctors. As geographer Mary Beth Pudup has argued, before the arrival of industrial capitalism in Appalachia, no significant markets existed for the skills of educated physicians.[13]

But some trained physicians did practice in preindustrial Appalachia. Before the economic expansion associated with the coal industry reshaped Appalachian life, locals negotiated their medical needs with physicians who possessed varying levels of formal education. Some physicians secured medical degrees by completing several years of didactic training and gaining clinical experience in an urban hospital. Others attended one or two sessions of medical lectures and served under a preceptor. A final group placed themselves under the tutelage of an established physician and never secured any formal medical education.[14] Such discrepancy in training,

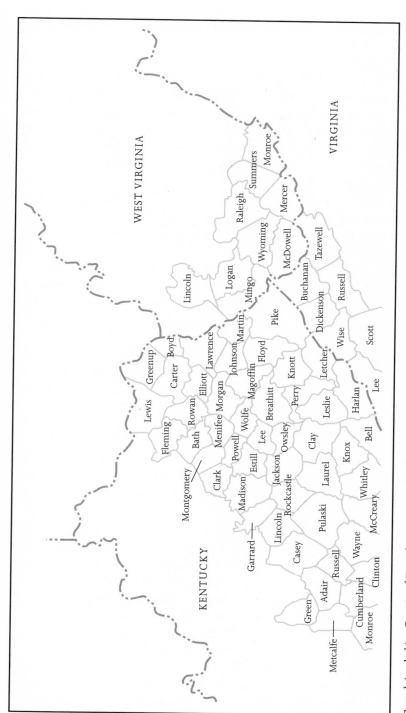

Central Appalachian Counties of Kentucky, Virginia, and West Virginia

William Rothstein and Thomas Bonner have argued, was typical in rural America.[15]

For Francis Fry of southwestern Virginia, attending a course of lectures at the Medical Department of Hampden-Sydney College in the winter of 1842 and working under a preceptor entitled him to return to southwestern Virginia and take up the practice of medicine. Students sometimes returned for a second course of lectures but most often completed only one course and then fulfilled the obligations set for them by their preceptor, obligations that were not always overseen by the medical school.[16]

The education offered at Hampden-Sydney's Medical Department was typical of that available at other regional medical schools across the country in the 1840s and 1850s.[17] Students were encouraged to embrace principles of observation and empirical evaluation, and Dr. John Cullen, who taught medical practice, "advocated and used freely the lancet, calomel, and opium." The catalog praised the school's lecture halls, dissecting room, and laboratories, but admission standards were low and full payment of fees typically guaranteed graduation.[18]

In 1854, infighting between faculty members and trustees led to the dissolution of the college's Medical Department and the creation of a new state-sponsored institution, the Medical College of Virginia. Few dramatic reforms were made, however, in admissions standards, the curriculum, or requirements for graduation. The Medical College of Virginia, like Hampden-Sydney, was the preferred school for men who sought the legitimacy bestowed by a formal medical education without having to incur the expense of journeying to a more established institution in another part of the country.

As such, the Medical College of Virginia became, and remained into the twentieth century, one of the most attractive institutions for Appalachian medical students, especially for those from Virginia and later West Virginia.[19] The college, however, was not unique in either its curriculum or its popularity among potential Appalachian physicians. The University of Louisville Medical Department, founded in 1845, and the College of Physicians and Surgeons in Baltimore, established in 1872, also educated a significant number of Appalachian physicians.[20]

The University of Louisville, the Medical College of Virginia, and the College of Physicians and Surgeons all struggled to support themselves on student fees.[21] In attempting to pay their bills and maintain faculty, these institutions, following the practices of other medical schools of the era, accepted most applicants and even negotiated with potential students the fees they would pay.[22] A young man from southwestern Virginia wrote to the dean of the Medical College of Virginia to request "a catalogue of the grand institution erected for the good of the human race. And the glory of god, not only in this world but in the world to come." While he gushed with enthusiasm about the college, he made it clear in his letter of 26 September 1886 that he was "going to attend some medical institution this coming winter and want[ed] to make preparations for starting at once."[23]

I. G. Haller, who completed the summer course at the Medical College of Virginia in 1870, wrote the college's dean, Levin Joynes, to request the "best arrangements you can negotiate for us in regards to professors' tickets, etc." To entice the dean to lower the price of admission for lectures and clinicals, Haller offered to bring other young men from his neighborhood who "speak of attending medical school this Fall." Haller assured the dean that if he agreed to charge a lower group rate he could prevent these young men from enrolling at a competing school in Baltimore. He also attempted to evoke the dean's sympathy by informing him that he was having difficulty collecting fees from his patients, revealing that, having completed only one course of lectures, he was already practicing medicine.[24]

Attendance at medical lectures, no matter how brief they might have been, seemed to earn doctors some degree of legitimacy. Dr. J. D. Kincaid, who began practicing in southwestern Virginia in 1843 and relocated to Catlettsburg, Kentucky, in 1847, only bothered to secure his first state medical license in 1893 when the state revamped its licensing procedures. His qualifications were fifty years of practice and attendance at one course of lectures at Jefferson Medical College in Philadelphia in the 1840s. Dr. J. S. Park, who practiced in Breathitt County, Kentucky, after relocating from Virginia in 1874, based his medical knowledge on his completion of one course of lectures at the Hospital College of Medicine in Richmond.[25]

In addition to the regional institutions, Jefferson Medical College was one of a number of other schools whose graduates practiced in the mountains of Appalachia before the expansion of the coal economy. Before the Civil War, physicians who claimed degrees from the University of Liverpool, the University of Pennsylvania, the University of Maryland, Transylvania University, and the University of Virginia as well as Jefferson Medical College and regional schools such as the Kentucky School of Medicine provided health care to Appalachian mountaineers. From 1865 until 1880, they were joined by graduates from the Eclectic Medical College of Louisville, the Medical College of Ohio, the Homeopathic Hospital College of Ohio, Miami Medical College, the College of Physicians and Surgeons in Baltimore, and the Cincinnati College of Physicians and Surgeons.[26]

Along with these graduates, many nondegreed physicians who had attended no medical courses at all also practiced in the mountains. When West Virginia began licensing doctors in the 1880s, it made provisions to grandfather in those who did not satisfy the new educational requirements but who had been practicing in the state for ten years or more. The state board of health's records indicate that 49.5 percent of those who were licensed at this time held no medical degree.[27]

Having acquired their training through apprenticeship or as autodidacts, many of these physicians were barely literate and occupied a unique position between lay healers and formally educated physicians. Neither of the two physicians listed in the 1870 census of Logan County, West Virginia, for example, identified themselves to the census taker as literate men.[28] Local history describes Dr. Emanual Church of southern West Virginia as "a typical mountaineer, uneducated and hardly able to read and write." He served his apprenticeship under Dr. C. J. Crockett of Wytheville, Virginia, who also acted as a preceptor for students from the Medical College of Virginia.[29]

Dr. Benjamin Hatton, who applied for a state license to practice medicine in Hazelgreen, Kentucky, in 1893, based his petition on thirty years of medical practice in the state. He noted that he was a graduate of "no school" on his application. Other physicians such as S. M. Ferguson, Charles Brian, Jesse Sturgell, and G. W. Wheeler, all of whom had begun to practice medicine in the Appalachian Mountains in the 1840s and 1850s, secured licenses although they had not attended a medical college, apparently acquiring their knowledge from preceptors.[30]

A letter from Dr. A. J. Robards to Kentucky governor Simon Buckner illustrates the lack of formal education of some physicians as well as their standing in the community. It also reveals the frontierlike nature of life in some corners of the Appalachians in the last decades of the nineteenth century. Writing to the governor in the midst of the French-Eversole feud in 1889, Robards expressed his frustration that the "good sciticins" of Breathitt, Perry, and Letcher Counties were unable to "pass up and down our county rodes with out bean shot at from the bresh." Robards's appeal demonstrates the deficiency of his formal education, but his belief that he spoke for the "good sciticins" of the county and his presumption that he could reasonably request personal aid from the governor suggest that, although poorly educated by abstract standards, he held a high position in the community.[31]

Community standing was as critical in defining a physician's status as education or philosophy of practice. In a history of the Big Sandy River valley between Kentucky and West Virginia written in 1887, William Ely categorized local physicians not by their educational background but by their family connections and the supplemental economic activities they pursued. Dr. S. M. Ferguson, whose application for a medical license indicated that he had never received formal education in the field, was described as the son-in-law of a judge and therefore "one of the prominent physicians in the Sandy Valley." As noted above, Dr. J. D. Kincaid, who Ely believed had the largest practice in the valley, acquired his medical training after completing one set of lectures at Jefferson Medical College. Dr. Allen Banfield, whose pedigree Ely explored thoroughly, came from a family of farmers, judges, capitalists, and physicians. Ely predicted that Banfield, although "at home in financial affairs," would continue to practice medicine instead of seeking public office, which someone in his position was expected to do; he preferred "to dictate good men to fill official stations [rather] than to hold them himself."[32]

Many physicians achieved economic, social, or political prominence, but many more were not so successful. Letters written by former and potential students to the dean of the Medical College of Virginia reveal that the pursuit of medicine alone did not guarantee one's economic status. In December 1869, Dr. I. M. Repass of southwestern Virginia wrote the dean about the $100 debt that he owed the college for a course he had completed in 1862. He explained that he had lost everything in the "late war" and that his medical practice did not provide him with enough income to fulfill his obligations. "The practice of medicine is not paying me, and I do not know how long I will remain."[33]

His sentiments were echoed by Dr. I. G. Haller, who complained that he found it "almost impossible to make collections."[34] Drs. R. A. Atkins and T. M. Painter, who also attended the Medical College of Virginia, were pursued by the school in 1870 for financial obligations they had incurred in 1868. The college employed William Terry, an attorney in Wytheville, Virginia, to collect the debts.[35]

In part, physicians of this era found it difficult to secure patients or successfully collect fees because they possessed relatively few remedies. In the years before Robert Koch and Louis Pasteur, physicians were trapped between the decline of heroic medicine and a growing reliance on the notion of specificity and the development of scientific medical therapies.[36] The few remaining records of Appalachian physicians' beliefs about medical therapeutics indicate that, like the physicians John Harley Warner has evaluated, they were facing a fundamental shift in their understanding of how to explain and treat illness.[37]

Events in 1835 in Lancaster, Kentucky, a community on the border between the eastern Kentucky mountains and the Bluegrass, confirm Warner's assertion that physicians were gradually moving away from reliance on heroic measures and toward more cautious treatments. The debate over appropriate therapies in this situation also illustrates generational tensions and the importance of recognizing the social context in which medicine is practiced.

Faced with a widespread outbreak of "fever," physicians struggled to determine both its origin and appropriate therapies. Many doctors insisted that the fever was caused by a "poisonous gas" that had been released by grading in the public square. This claim, however, was challenged by other physicians not because they dismissed the dangers of miasmatic air but because they believed the weather was too cold for the disease to have been dispersed in this fashion. Those who rejected the poisonous gas theory insisted that a nearby pond and swamp had produced the disease. Dr. Luther Buford, a Transylvania University graduate who wrote about the case in his alma mater's medical journal, argued that "the malaria arising from this filthy spot had some agency in producing the scarlet fever of 1831, dysentery of 1832, cholera in 1833, and the disease of which I am treating."[38]

Buford also disagreed with his colleagues over the appropriate remedy for the malady. Older physicians in the community "excited public prejudices against the use of the lancet," but Buford wrote that, if he were unfettered to practice as he chose, he would "bleed again and again." His statement supports Warner's argument that although heroic medicine was fading from vogue, physicians still believed that bleeding had a place in the therapeutic arsenal.[39]

Buford was not free to follow his own convictions in this case, however, because of his "youthful appearance and want of experience." He regretted his failure to pursue the treatment he desired and vowed that in the future "he would not allow [his] timidity and deference for the mere opinions of men of experience to induce [him] to neglect the employment of a remedy of so much importance." Although convinced of the medical virtues of his planned cure, he was prevented from administering it by the social environment in which he practiced.[40]

Other records document the slow transformation of medical knowledge among Appalachian physicians in the nineteenth century. As late as 1890, physicians in Bell County, Kentucky, were explaining episodes of ill health in Middlesboro as a consequence of "miasmatic influence."[41] Early physicians who practiced on the West Virginia side of the Tug River valley during the 1860s and 1870s revealed their allegiance to heroic treatments by relying on cathartics to empty the bowels and restore the body's equilibrium. Like other physicians in the era, they also increasingly turned to the use of alcohol and "blood thinning" to soothe distressed patients.[42] The persistence of such beliefs does not indicate that Appalachian physicians were reluctant to embrace new scientific presumptions; instead, it demonstrates that, like many rural physicians across the United States, Appalachian doctors had yet to acquire a full comprehension of the new scientific advances that were redefining medical practice.[43]

Doubly burdened by the general immaturity of medical science and the inadequate training of mountain physicians, who did not possess even the meager knowledge claimed by urban physicians, rural mountain residents continued to rely on a rich tradition of folk healing throughout the nineteenth century. Many mountain residents possessed little or no knowledge of the practices of modern medicine. "A doctor," wrote mountain native Emma Bell Miles in the early twentieth century, "is not thought of."[44] As late as the mid-twentieth century, lifetime residents of isolated mountain settlements recalled that few physicians had ever visited their rural homes and that traveling to a doctor's office was even more rare.[45]

Many rural Appalachian residents drew on folklore or their contact with Native Americans for relief from illness or pain.[46] Local "witch doctors," as they were sometimes described by outside observers, served rural populations by preparing herbal remedies and offering charms.[47] These healers shared the assumption of their patients, who were also their neighbors, that illness was a reflection of an imbalance within the body and that purges and other medicines that altered the body's temperature could restore equilibrium, an assumption that revealed the intrusion of heroic notions of illness and therapy into this isolated region.[48] Mountain folklore also celebrated mystical cures and magical spells. The importance of these remedies was demonstrated in the 1820s when a compilation of magical cures entitled *John George Hohman's Pow-Wows* was translated from the original German and published in English. According to anthropologist Joan Moser, this work was commonly found in households from Pennsylvania to eastern Kentucky and served as a critical reference for many Appalachian people.[49] Even in recent decades, mountaineers have expressed strong beliefs in magical cures and the healing power of prayer.[50]

Religious faith also influenced the attitudes of mountaineers toward pain and illness. Miles observed that Appalachian people who lived outside settled areas seldom sought medical assistance because most illnesses were "endured as a matter of course."[51] When a public health nurse in eastern Kentucky encouraged a father to allow his children to have their tonsils removed, he replied, "The Lord giveth and the Lord taketh away. Blessed be the name of the Lord. The children's tonsils shall not be removed."[52] Prayer also played a pivotal role in guiding healers in their efforts to cure the afflicted.[53]

In her novella *Sight to the Blind*, Lucy Furman, a twentieth-century settlement worker in Kentucky, insisted that highlanders were fatalistic and averse to new therapies and treatments. Furman's book related the story of an elderly woman who believed that her blindness was divine punishment for the sin of blasphemy. Ridden by guilt and hopelessness, she refused to pursue medical treatment until a public health nurse from a local settlement school convinced her that there was a physiological rather than a theological explanation for her handicap. After leaving her community for successful treatment, the elderly woman returned a new champion of modern medicine.[54]

In spite of the fatalism described in *Sight to the Blind* and reinforced by Miles and other writers such as John C. Campbell, rural mountain residents did not irrationally reject medical care.[55] Rising poverty and landlessness in the nineteenth century burdened rural mountaineers, but, like the family of Jane Crawford, who transported her sixty miles so she could undergo an experimental surgical procedure, country people vigorously pursued innovative cures when they were available.[56] As an impoverished people spread across a daunting landscape, rural Appalachian residents could not easily secure the skills of educated physicians. Prayer, folk healing, stoicism, and tenacity were free or could be acquired locally through barter; trained doctors seldom lived nearby, and their services were expensive. Mountain poverty and isolation, not tradition, prevented Appalachian residents from obtaining medical care.

Mountaineers demonstrated their willingness to seek affordable medical relief through their growing attachment for patent medicines, an attachment they shared with other rural Americans. Like farmers and country people elsewhere, Appalachians saw these remedies as effective yet inexpensive cures.[57] Panaceas like oil for earaches and salves for chest ailments became increasingly popular throughout the mountains during this era.[58]

The reputation and economic significance of these tonics became so great that the state of West Virginia initiated court cases against itinerant vendors who sold "drugs or nostrums" without paying the appropriate tax. When J. B. Ragland began selling Ragland's Lightening Relief for fifty cents a bottle in Boone County, West Virginia, in 1887, he found a receptive market among the poorer residents of the county. The local sheriff, however, discovered that Ragland had failed to pay the "special tax" levied on this type of commercial activity and arrested him. Ragland's arrest and conviction were eventually upheld by the West Virginia Court of Appeals, and Ragland was forced to pay the assessed penalties and taxes.[59] Taxing patent medicines benefited doctors and druggists who resided in towns and who sought to advance their own status by discouraging selfhealing and self-medication. For mountaineers, the regulation of patent medicines removed a familiar remedy from their home medicine cabinets.

The increased visibility of patent medicine vendors, as well as the state's drive to limit such sales, symbolized the commercial growth of the region associated with the arrival of large-scale timber and coal-mining operations.[60] As the old order was replaced by economic relationships characteristic of advanced capitalism, many mountain people lost the ability to secure their livelihood through agriculture or small-scale commercial production.[61] With the creation of company timber and coal-mining villages, the region was transformed by the arrival of tens of thousands of European immigrants and African Americans escaping the Deep South in search of greater civil liberties. They joined Appalachian residents who were forced to give up land to speculators or who willingly accepted wage work in the industrial sector.[62]

In the *First Annual Report of the State Inspector of Mines* issued in 1884, the government of West Virginia documented the existence of only sixty-three mines in the southern portion of the state. These mines produced about 1.5 million tons of coal and employed 4,162 miners. The employment opportunities were important for local residents, but coal mining was not yet a pivotal economic enterprise for the state. Most of the coal mines were situated in Fayette and Kanawha Counties along the Kanawha River, indicating the industry's reliance on traditional methods of transportation and settlement.[63] By the turn of the century, however, conditions had changed dramatically and coal had become a principal component of West Virginia's economy as industrialists used newly constructed railroads to transport coal from the previously isolated areas of southern West Virginia.

Similar transformations occurred later in Virginia and eastern Kentucky.[64] Coal was first commercially mined in southwestern Virginia in 1882, but it was only after the turn of the century that output skyrocketed and counties such as Wise and Tazewell became centers of large-scale commercial production.[65] The expansion of the Kentucky coal industry in the first decades of the twentieth century as some of the richest coal deposits in the Appalachians were discovered and exploited continued the gradual transformation of the region.[66]

As industrial production of coal and timber soared, the number of workers employed in these industries rose dramatically. From 1900 to 1910, coal mines in McDowell County, West Virginia, increased their workforce from 6,311 to over 16,000. Raleigh County, West Virginia, officials reported a tenfold increase in the number of miners employed in their county during the same era.[67] During its period of greatest growth, eastern Kentucky experienced an equally astonishing rise in the number of men employed in the mining industry.[68] Similar increases occurred in the coal mines of southwestern Virginia.[69]

As mining expanded, new towns were formed and previously existing villages quickly grew in size. The population of Bluefield, West Virginia, increased from 1,775 in 1890 to over 11,000 in 1910. Beckley, West Virginia, expanded from a village of 158 in

1890 to a community of over 2,000 twenty years later. Williamson and Scarbro, West Virginia, not incorporated in 1890, each had over 1,000 inhabitants by 1910.[70] Eastern Kentucky and southwestern Virginia experienced a similar rise in both population and the number of towns.[71]

Those who accepted industrialists' offers of employment in the coal mines of Central Appalachia found themselves engaged in dangerous work. In 1909–10, more than 100 miners were killed in accidents in McDowell County, West Virginia, 60 died in Fayette County, and 19 died in Raleigh County. Nonfatal injuries were even more prevalent. In McDowell County, 246 men suffered nonfatal accidents, and in Fayette County, 213 men were injured in mining mishaps during the same period.[72] To encourage people to undertake such dangerous work and to prevent a decrease in production due to injury or sickness, companies hired physicians to oversee the welfare of their workers. These young doctors, as well as their colleagues who set up private practices in growing Appalachian towns, heralded the scientific advances gradually being introduced into their medical school curricula.

On the surface, it might appear that company owners employed doctors for essentially benign reasons. Many of the coal camps were simply too remote to attract physicians seeking to set up independent private practices, so operators attempted to aid their workers by providing trained physicians.[73] But mine owners were also determined to limit the amount of work lost by miners who were injured on the job. Like their efforts to reduce the possibility of explosions or cave-ins, owners' efforts to protect the health of their workers were based on their concerns about the economic as well as the human costs of injury or death.[74]

Proximity to an educated physician was also an attractive draw to entice workers into the coal camps. For rural Appalachians who moved into mining villages, the presence of an educated doctor was a benefit of town life previously unavailable to them. African Americans who had faced Jim Crow in the Deep South welcomed the opportunity to receive competent medical care.[75] Engaged in a dangerous enterprise, miners and their families were comforted to know that a physician lived nearby. "Labor was scarce," according to coal archivist Stuart McGehee, "and trained doctors were an incentive to attract good miners."[76]

Operators were also happy to have the companionship of educated practitioners.[77] As members of a fledgling profession that consciously worked to improve its social status and public powers, physicians became important allies in the operators' campaigns to create a new middle class that depended on the economic activity of the coalfields for stability.[78] As such, doctors promised to improve the lives of their patients in return for appropriate deference to their professional skills.[79] Offering a "prophecy of progress," educated doctors, like other agents of industrial capitalism, pledged to reward miners who accepted the new rules that ordered life both in the mines and outside them.[80]

The opportunities offered by the expansion of the medical market initially were made available to physicians who were already in residence when the railroads, the first overt sign of capital's intrusion, came to the mountains. Physicians who had acquired formal medical training and whose families were already part of the local elite found themselves in an advantageous position, able to secure employment from railroad, timber, or coal companies or to expand their private practices in the growing towns of Central Appalachia.[81]

Elliot Rutherford was born in southwestern Virginia during "pioneer days," and his family owned land in the Tug River valley throughout the nineteenth century. The son of Scottish immigrants, Rutherford attended Cincinnati Medical College and practiced medicine in Mingo County, West Virginia, where he also farmed and operated a small timbering operation. He served as a surgeon for the Confederate forces during the Civil War. His son Lewis Rutherford was a farmer, a sawmill operator, and the owner of more than 2,300 acres of coal land. Three of Lewis Rutherford's sons were physicians like their grandfather; two of them relocated to "Indian territory," but the oldest of the three, Albert, stayed behind to make his fortune in southern West Virginia. Four years of teaching in the public schools provided Albert Rutherford with the savings to attend the University of Tennessee Medical School in Nashville, where he received his medical degree in 1900. He obtained employment at a coal company in which his family had interests and as a physician for the Norfolk and Western Railroad, which was being constructed through the region to transport coal from the Tug River valley. Along with his company employment, Rutherford continued his family's tradition of community and political involvement, serving in both public and private capacities.[82]

Family ties also facilitated the professional lives of Isaiah Bee and his son, Isaiah Ernest Bee, of Princeton, West Virginia. The grandson of a Revolutionary War soldier, the elder Bee grew up on the family's land grant in northwestern Virginia. After studying under a physician for two years, he attended medical lectures in Cleveland and began practicing medicine in 1859. Upon completion of his service in the Confederate army, he opened a practice in Mercer County in southern West Virginia. In addition to his medical endeavors, he was a member of the state's Constitutional Convention and a state representative for many years. Although Bee never worked as a company doctor, he invested in coal operations and was a great civic and commercial booster for Princeton. The younger Bee, Isaiah Ernest, began his medical practice in 1890, in the middle of the initial coal boom in southern West Virginia. A graduate of the College of Physicians and Surgeons in Baltimore, Bee maintained a private practice but also served as a physician for the Virginia Railway.[83]

Like the Bee family, the Farleys, who lived on both sides of the Tug River in Kentucky and West Virginia, used family ties, physical proximity to sites of economic development, and education to secure their economic and social status in the evolving political economy. William Farley was the oldest of five brothers who all became coal company physicians. Born in Pike County, Kentucky, in 1866, he later taught school across the Tug River in Logan County, West Virginia, for ten years. In 1893, after graduating from the Medical College of the University of Louisville, he established a private practice in Logan. When the U.S. Coal and Oil Company was organized there in 1903, he invested in the corporation and became its surgeon, overseeing the medical care of its employees. He also served as president of the county court for many years, following in the footsteps of his father, who had been a justice of the peace and a county assessor.[84]

Another example of a physician who built on family ties to assure his position in the industrial economy was Henry D. Hatfield. Henry Hatfield, a nephew of Devil Anse Hatfield, followed his father into Logan County politics as well as pursuing a medical degree. Although popular myth has depicted the Hatfields as infamous hillbillies, Altina Waller has argued convincingly that many of their difficulties arose from their efforts to improve their economic status in the new commercial economy. Henry Hatfield's career illustrates the success of one branch of the family in achieving social, economic, and political prestige. After completing his medical degree, he became chief surgeon of the state-sponsored Miners' Hospital No. 1 in Welch, West Virginia. Along with his position at the hospital, he served as a physician for as many as nine coal companies at a time, although he turned those practices over to an assistant when he was elected governor of West Virginia in 1912.[85]

The Rutherfords, Bees, Farleys, and Hatfields were already well positioned when representatives of outside industrial concerns arrived in Appalachia to build railroads and buy up timber and mineral rights. As members of the region's preindustrial elite who also possessed formal medical credentials, they were empowered to negotiate between the established order and the new industrial interests. For Appalachian physicians who lacked ties to the established elite or the credentials necessary to prosper in the developing political economy, however, the benefits of the region's expanding economy were less easily secured.

Dr. Emanual Church, who possessed only empirical medical training and was essentially illiterate, saw his practice vanish in McDowell County, West Virginia, when "the coal companies opened up and the company doctors arrived." He relocated to the mountains of Greenbrier and Pocahontas Counties, in a less settled, less industrialized section of southeastern West Virginia, where he continued his practice. Dr. Hiram Christian, like Church, closed his practice when competition for patients became too intense. Rather than resettle in a more isolated area, however, he changed careers, opening a law office in Welch, West Virginia. Finding the legal profession too crowded in the county seat, he eventually moved to War, where he became justice of the peace.[86] Dr. H. F. Neel, who established a practice in Tazewell, Virginia, left that area when the coal industry began to restructure the local political economy. He moved to Pike County, Kentucky, later abandoning his practice there when the local coalfields were opened for development and new doctors moved into the area.[87]

Many members of the earlier generation of Appalachian physicians gave up and left their practices, but others persisted and continued to be patronized by mountain residents who lived outside mining and timbering camps. Mountaineers who were not yet fully invested in the cash economy that was gaining ground across the coal region relied on these older doctors in part because they shared rural residents' comfort with the barter system. Like the West Virginians Ronald L. Lewis has described who moved with ease between the subsistence economy and the cash economy, doctors often accepted compensation in produce or manual labor as well as in cash.[88]

Accustomed to relating to their healers as members of their own communities, rural mountain people often failed to fully comprehend younger physicians' desire for immediate cash compensation. Some doctors resorted to harsh tactics to teach patients their proper role in the economic relationship that supported modern medicine. A southern West Virginia physician, summoned to examine the children of an isolated mountain family, discovered that they had been exposed to diphtheria and that one of the children was already exhibiting symptoms. The doctor, who had brought with him the appropriate antitoxin, "refused to administer the medicine unless he was paid $60 in advance."[89] In his book Coal Towns, Crandall Shifflet related the story of a mountain family in Knott County, Kentucky, who lost their farm to a doctor who foreclosed on it when they were unable to pay the $300 medical bill a dying grandparent had accumulated.[90]

Early industrial workers who were still intimately tied to traditional mountain life also questioned the imposition of a new economic structure to support health care.[91] Company employees, willing to accept many of the advantages and obligations of wage employment, sometimes rejected requirements that they help finance the retention of a physician through the checkoff system, whereby their contributions were automatically deducted from their wages. In protest, one group of miners engaged in a spontaneous public theater in which they feigned illness in order to acquire drugs from the physician and then discarded the medicine as useless, insisting that the doctor offered only "soda and flour."[92]

Native mountaineers might have found the transition to modern medical care more palatable if resident physicians had controlled it, but the dramatic increase in population in Central Appalachia attracted an enormous number of new doctors to the region. This new opportunity for physicians conveniently arose at the same time that the medical marketplace was flooded by physicians who were graduating from the plethora of proprietary schools created after the Civil War.[93] In search of stable employment and opportunities to develop private practices, physicians from outside the mountains, as well as ambitious locals, sought to secure their livelihoods in coal camps or in growing communities nearby. As table 1.1 indicates, the arrival of these new physicians significantly increased the number of physicians practicing in the mountains between 1886 and 1917.

Besides this increase in number, the medical population also underwent a shift in composition. Polk's Medical Register and Directory of the United States and Canada, which attempted to list all practicing physi-

Table 1.1 Number of Physicians in Central Appalachian Sections of
Kentucky, Virginia, and West Virginia, 1886–1917

Year	Kentucky	Virginia	West Virginia
1886	77	105	40
1896	176	124	103
1906	229	112	233
1917	234	121	281

Sources: Polk, *Medical and Surgical Directory*, 1886, *Medical and Surgical Register*, 1896,
Medical Register, 1906, 1917; Ronald Eller, *Miners, Millhands, and Mountaineers*,
150–52.

cians, relied on the doctors themselves to supply information on their medical degrees. The changes in the data they provided over the decades demonstrate the evolving profile of the medical profession in Central Appalachia. It would be erroneous to assume that all of the physicians who failed to report their degrees were uneducated, but the rise in the number of physicians who did embrace this type of promotion suggests a growing interest in the advancement of the medical profession through such modern devices as advertising. The percentages of physicians who reported their degree information between 1886 and 1917 are presented in table 1.2.

Table 1.3 shows the rise in the number of medical schools reportedly attended by physicians who practiced in Central Appalachia between 1886 and 1917. As graduates from a growing assortment of schools moved into the region, they brought with them a diversity of experience and education that had not existed among earlier doctors in the mountains. Physicians educated at elite institutions had a greater knowledge of the laboratory sciences than did their colleagues who held less prestigious degrees. Doctors who had matriculated at second- or third-tier institutions in other parts of the nation found themselves competing for positions with locals who enjoyed established ties and other outsiders who had more impressive credentials. Possessing varied backgrounds, these newcomers were bound together by little besides their professional identity.

The rise in the number of physicians reporting degrees and in the variety of schools from which they graduated contributes to the development of a portrait of the new physicians who invaded the Appalachians at the end of the nineteenth century. This portrait is enhanced by a consideration of the years in which doctors received their degrees. Such an analysis reveals that more recently graduated

Table 1.2 Percentage of Physicians in Central Appalachian Sections of Kentucky, Virginia, and West Virginia Reporting Medical Degrees to Polk's *Medical Register,* 1886–1917

Year	Kentucky	Virginia	West Virginia
1886	19	9	45
1896	43	42	69
1906	62	62	69
1917	93	95	99

Sources: Polk, *Medical and Surgical Directory,* 1886, *Medical and Surgical Register,* 1896, *Medical Register,* 1906, 1917.

physicians were moving into the mountains, not that more resident physicians were reporting to the *Medical Register.*

It was apparent even in 1886 that more recently educated physicians were making headway in Appalachia. In that year, 47 percent of physicians reporting degrees in Kentucky, 44 percent in Virginia, and 61 percent in West Virginia had earned them in the preceding decade. By 1896, 81 percent of the Kentuckians who reported degrees, 56 percent of the Virginians, and 72 percent of the West Virginians had graduated between 1886 and 1895.

By 1906, the percentages of practicing physicians who earned degrees between 1886 and 1905 clearly demonstrated the generational and educational shift that expedited the transformation of medicine in the mountains. Physicians who reported in 1906 that they had earned degrees between 1896 and 1905 were 29, 30, and 36 percent of those who reported degrees in Kentucky, Virginia, and West Virginia, respectively. Combining these figures with the percentages of those who had received degrees between 1886 and 1895 reveals that 50 percent of the Kentucky physicians reporting degrees, 46 percent of the Virginia doctors, and 55 percent of those practicing in West Virginia earned their diplomas between 1886 and 1905.[94]

The number of physicians practicing in Central Appalachia rose dramatically from 222 in 1886 to 403 in 1896. Of those who reported to Polk in 1886, 58, or just over 26 percent, indicated that they possessed medical degrees. Ten years later, 201, or 50 percent, supplied Polk with information about their medical degrees. More than 33 percent of all physicians practicing in Central Appalachia in 1896 and more than 70 percent of those reporting degrees had graduated between 1886 and 1895.[95]

Table 1.3 Number of Medical Schools Attended by Physicians in Central Appalachian Sections of Kentucky, Virginia, and West Virginia, 1886–1917

Year	Kentucky	Virginia	West Virginia
1886	11	10	10
1896	19	16	23
1906	27	19	38
1917	37	27	47

Sources: Polk, *Medical and Surgical Directory*, 1886, *Medical and Surgical Register*, 1896, *Medical Register*, 1906, 1917.

The number of physicians continued to rise from 1896 to 1917, although in a less dramatic fashion. By 1906, 574 doctors were practicing in the region; of the 66 percent who reported possessing diplomas, 49 percent had acquired their degrees in the previous ten years. By 1917, the increase had tapered off significantly as medical schools closed in the face of educational reforms and the number of new physicians declined nationally.[96]

Many of the young physicians practicing medicine in Central Appalachia in these critical decades were, like Isaiah Ernest Bee, the Farley brothers, and Henry Hatfield, locals who had left the mountains to secure medical training. Others, however, were outsiders who came to Appalachia seeking economic opportunity. An evaluation of membership records of the West Virginia State Medical Association reveals that of 192 physicians who enrolled in the association from the relevant counties from 1900 to 1925, 71, or 37 percent, were from outside the region.[97]

Many newcomers were brought to the Appalachian coalfields by friends and colleagues from medical school. Through a type of collegial chain migration, mountaineers who attended medical schools in Louisville and Richmond introduced their classmates to the economic rewards available in the coal camps and boomtowns of the region. After graduation, professional contact between those who practiced in the mountains and those who did not created ongoing opportunities for local doctors to spread the good news of Appalachia's economic development.

Dr. J. B. Bartram moved to southern West Virginia and established his practice in the mining camp at Dingess in Mingo County after his graduation from the University of Louisville in 1891. A year later, his classmate, Dr. L. T. Loar, followed him. After Drs. O. J. Henderson and William Klase completed their training at the Medical College of Virginia in 1889, they both relocated to Montgomery, West Virginia. Dr. L. D. Rupert graduated from the University of Louisville in 1892; his classmate Dr. J. Wallis Walker joined him in Winona, where they provided medical care for the coal miners who worked in the area and their families.[98]

After William Price of Virginia finished his medical education at the University of Virginia, the same institution from which his father and brother had graduated, he followed his older brother into the coalfields of southern West Virginia. Drs. Luther Clark and William Thomas graduated in 1892 from the College of Physicians and Surgeons in Baltimore. Although they were West Virginians, neither of them had been reared in the coal-producing regions of the state. Upon graduation, however, they settled in the southern part of West Virginia and took up coal and railroad practices.[99]

Employment by an industrial concern provided a steady income, but it did not guarantee long-term success, and young physicians struggled to secure their position in the growing Appalachian economy. Dr. Woods, a young outsider who served as the company doctor for the Ritter Lumber Company, provided medical care in the Dry Fork and Panther Creek regions of southern West Virginia from 1900 to 1907. When the company completed its cutting in the region, he moved on to the next job site with the rest of the workers. Dr. Septimus Kell, a 1907 graduate of the College of Physicians and Surgeons in Baltimore, signed on as the physician for the Lathrop Coal Company in 1913. After supervising the health care of the population of the four mining camps that comprised Lathrop's operations, Kell eventually left the area around 1926. Even a native as well connected as Dr. S. D. Hatfield, a son of Devil Anse Hatfield who graduated from the University of Louisville in 1906, faced uncertainty when he opened a medical practice in Iaeger, West Virginia, in 1907. He remained in the community until 1920 but departed after timber companies completed their work because travel on the poorly maintained roads was difficult and the local people had little money to spend on medical care.[100]

The isolation of the coal camps and the boom-and-bust cycle of coal production made for an uncertain economic future for many company physicians. A brief survey of the history of the medical practitioners who served several mining communities demonstrates the ephemeral nature of some physicians' tenure. In 1896, no formally trained physicians practiced in Big Stone Gap, Virginia. Ten years later, 1,000 people resided there, and four educated physicians tended to their needs. The town's population doubled in the next decade, but the number of physicians was cut in half since all of the previous providers, with the exception of Dr. James Kelly, had relocated. Kelly had been joined by a recent graduate. In 1917, the town's population had grown to 2,590, and four physicians practiced there.[101]

Big Stone Gap was a commercial center as well as being tied to the coal industry. In communities more dependent on coal, the economic instability of medical practitioners was more marked. Drs. Bartram and Loar, who had moved to Dingess, West Virginia, after graduating from the University of Louisville in the early 1890s, had both relocated by 1906. The two physicians who had taken their place had also abandoned the town by 1917. Ansted, West Virginia, boasted no physicians in 1886, but four doctors practiced there in 1896, two of whom were recent graduates of the University of Louisville. Ten years later, three of the four doctors had relocated, including both of the Louisville graduates, and they had been replaced by two recent graduates. By 1917, an entirely new complement of physicians served Ansted.[102] Ronald Lewis, in his recent work on timbering in the West Virginia backcountry, has documented the same instability among medical practitioners in timbering villages.[103]

Uncertain about their ability to secure a reasonable income from their medical practices, some physicians pursued alternative or related endeavors to augment their income. A number responded to the growing demand for specialized services by opening hospitals that supplemented their incomes while providing the community with inpatient facilities. Dr. John T. Graham, for example, constructed a hospital in Wytheville, Virginia, in 1899 that catered to the women of the growing town elite who sought medical care during childbirth.[104] Other physicians scrambled to acquire government positions at state institutions or as county public health administrators, a reflection of the government's increasing reliance on trained doctors as well as physicians' desire to acquire a secure income.[105]

Although all of these strategies improved a physician's chances of achieving success, many outside physicians found that forming professional and personal alliances with entrenched locals greatly increased their prospects. Dr. J. Frank Fox, a North Carolina native, was

Bringing Modern Medicine to the Mountains

the son of a physician. A graduate of the University of Virginia who completed his medical degree at New York University, Fox established his first practice in the community of Waynesboro, Virginia, in the Shenandoah Valley. This enterprise failed to prosper, however, and in 1892, he accepted a contract with the Norfolk and Western Railroad to care for its employees in the Pocahontas coalfield.[106]

Fox sought to expand his practice beyond railroad work and joined forces with a local physician, Dr. Wade St. Clair. A native of Tazewell County, Virginia, St. Clair had attended the University of Virginia's Medical College.[107] Fox and St. Clair established Bluefield, West Virginia's, first hospital in 1902, which eventually became one of the most modern institutions in the region.[108] When they decided to expand the facility in 1914, they took advantage of the financial success of St. Clair's father, a native industrialist who had profited from the region's development. Alexander St. Clair, who continued to reside on the family farm in Tazewell County, became a partner in the corporation that was established to fund the new facility.[109]

Dr. Wilkin B. Stevens possessed little other than his medical credentials when he moved to southern West Virginia in 1905. Raised in Milltown, Alabama, and forced to provide for his family at age twelve after his father died, Stevens paid for his own high school expenses and saved enough to enroll at Maryland Medical College in 1899, an institution Abraham Flexner described as "wretchedly dirty" and possessing laboratories "of the worst type."[110] After his graduation in 1904, he made his way to the coalfields of Central Appalachia, where he became an assistant company doctor. Given the quality of his medical training, Stevens might have had a career of little renown, but he caught the attention of Dr. Henry Hatfield and became his assistant at Miners' Hospital No. 1, a publicly funded emergency hospital in Welch, West Virginia. When Hatfield was elected governor of the state in 1912, Stevens took over his practices at nine mining operations; he also followed Hatfield onto the boards of several banks and was a loyal political supporter.[111]

By tying themselves to the established elite, newly arrived physicians attempted to solidify their position in the Appalachian middle class. Doctors also sought to improve their fortunes through connections with newly constructed institutions. By accepting positions as company doctors, seeking employment in state-sponsored facilities such as Miners' Hospital No. 1, and establishing private practices in growing communities, physicians who moved into Central Appalachia before the turn of the century sought to profit from the region's new prosperity.

Although determined to take advantage of the new commercial economy developing in the mountains, many physicians found their practices unstable and their economic futures uncertain. If they were unable to forge ties with the established elite or if they grew dissatisfied with their role as employees of coal or railroad companies, they had only a weak foundation on which to fall back. With the expansion of the economy and the rapid intrusion of new physicians into the region, doctors were vulnerable to market forces that could displace them. In order to protect themselves and guarantee their stability in the evolving economy, physicians had to capitalize on the economic expansion and create a professional identity that would unite physicians across the region.

CHAPTER TWO

Physicians

and the Quest

for Professional

Identity

The boomtowns and coal camps of Central Appalachia offered the young physicians who flocked to the region at the end of the nineteenth century more than employment. The positions they secured with industry provided immediate rewards, but many of these men recognized that the coalfields, so poorly served by trained physicians before industrialization, also gave them the opportunity to redefine their professional identity. These young physicians seized the occasion to consolidate their economic and social positions by joining with ambitious colleagues across the United States in a campaign to improve their occupational status by building on the scientific promises of the late nineteenth century.[1]

Most of the physicians who moved into the region shared the desire to secure increased professional prestige and social and economic status, but disharmony persisted concerning both the form and the content of medicine. Although doctors might unite in a campaign to gain recognition for their occupation, disparities in social standing, educational experience, and medical philosophy divided them. Reformers initiated a campaign to remake medical education in the late nineteenth century, but this crusade came late to schools that prepared mountain doctors, and inequality of training, acquisition of internship experience, and completion of graduate courses divided physicians into those who possessed extensive clinical and laboratory experience and those who did not.[2]

Over time, the homogenization of medical education advanced the trends that would eventually unite Appalachian physicians in a common educational experience. To further their professional connections, doctors also invested more time and resources in their private medical associations. These organizations became vehicles to promote self-regulation, encourage professional development, and oppose potential competitors who embraced alternative medical philosophies. Medical societies also lobbied for state licensing laws that favored "regular" healers and denied parity to sectarians.[3]

Physicians fostered close alliances with the state in order to maintain their advantage over their competitors. Possessing a near monopoly over the definition and practice of medicine, doctors could claim to be protecting the health of the public from the inept manipulations of sectarians. These aspiring professionals also sought to capitalize on their intimate ties with the state in other ways, seeking appointments to state and local boards of public health so that they could use those positions to displace older physicians who had conflicting presumptions about what defined medical authority and practice.[4]

Barbara Rosenkrantz, in writing about physicians who engaged in public health work before the last decades of the nineteenth century, has argued that "there was the clear sense that [a doctor's] contribution lay less in his scientific acumen than in his responsible citizenship."[5] As older doctors who took their identities from their community standing were replaced by younger physicians who had at least a rudimentary knowledge of bacteriology, new definitions of professional legitimacy and of the authority of the doctor in the community were created. These redefinitions were hastened by the intrusion of the state as officers of departments of public health arrived to speak for the virtues of new scientific principles in a voice that drowned out the protests of older physicians whose therapeutic beliefs, as well as the social and political systems under which they had practiced, were being stifled.[6]

Like older doctors, midwives were experiencing the fundamental redefinition of the world they and their foremothers had known for centuries. Unlike physicians, however, lay healers made no claim to the title of "professional" and were therefore more difficult targets for doctors seeking to redefine medical therapeutics and medical legitimacy. In spite of their best efforts to create a monopoly supported by the state, the new physicians who moved into Appalachia during industrialization faced formidable opposition from healers who made no assertion of professional identity.

Eliot Friedson has argued that possession of expert knowledge is the first pillar of professionalism. For Appalachian physicians, that expertise was a matter of some debate in the last decades of the nineteenth century. Younger physicians who held medical diplomas seemed to boast the most overt symbol of specialized knowledge, but the meaning behind that symbol was still being debated both inside and outside the medical community. As the lives of Appalachian residents were increasingly complicated by their entanglement in the market economy, they looked to medical professionals and the credentials they possessed to "narrow the range of choice," an undertaking physicians willingly pursued since it empowered those who possessed scientific knowledge to displace their competitors.[7]

The reform of the medical curriculum was a critical element in the construction of medical expertise at the end of the nineteenth century. As has been well documented, Harvard University, the University of Michigan, the University of Pennsylvania, and the newly established Johns Hopkins University led the way in medical reform in the last three decades of the century. By lengthening the university term, introducing a graded curriculum, elevating admissions standards, and requiring extensive laboratory training and clinical experience, these institutions began the development of the modern medical school. Such reform, however, had relatively little immediate impact on the schools typically attended by Appalachian physicians.[8]

Although the number of mountain doctors who held degrees rose sharply after 1885 and an increasingly wide array of schools were represented in the region, between one-third and one-half of the doctors who practiced in the area from 1885 to 1925 were educated at three institutions: the Medical College of Virginia, the University of Louisville, and the College of Physicians and Surgeons in Baltimore. These schools, while hardly the worst examples of proprietary colleges in existence, were slow to embrace reform.

A survey of 192 physicians in the southern coalfields who joined the West Virginia State Medical Association between 1900 and 1925 reveals that more than 23 percent were educated at the Medical College of Virginia, 15 percent at the University of Louisville, and over 8 percent at the College of Physicians and Surgeons in Baltimore. Almost 47 percent, therefore, were educated at these three schools.[9]

In 1906, Polk's Medical Register reported that nearly 13 percent of the degreed physicians across the region were educated at the Medical

College of Virginia, 12 percent at the University of Louisville, and more than 7 percent at the College of Physicians and Surgeons in Baltimore. Eleven years later, 13 percent of those with diplomas had attended the Medical College of Virginia, 20 percent the University of Louisville, and 11 percent the College of Physicians and Surgeons in Baltimore. When graduates of proprietary schools such as Maryland Medical College and the Kentucky School of Medicine, which were eventually subsumed by their stronger neighbors, are included, the totals indicate that the majority of Appalachian physicians were educated at regional institutions, especially those in Richmond, Louisville, and Baltimore.[10]

Students who attended schools such as these in the period from 1880 to 1910 received a very different education from that of students who attended elite institutions. Although much has been written about the reform of top-tier medical programs, little research has been done on the content of medical education at less prestigious medical institutions. As Charlotte Borst has demonstrated in her study of Wisconsin physicians, graduates of these institutions were more cognizant of the promises of science than they were of its practice.[11]

The Medical College of Virginia, founded in 1854, was popular among young southern men throughout the last half of the nineteenth century. As southern students abandoned northern schools to matriculate back home in Dixie during this period, the college enjoyed a stable enrollment. The school was attractive in part because admission and graduation were nearly assured to anyone who could pay the required tuition and fees.[12] Until the 1880s, the curriculum consisted of two years of lectures, the second being a repeat of the first. Admissions standards were low, if they existed at all. Access to clinical training was also a difficulty for Medical College of Virginia students in the nineteenth century since the college had no direct hospital affiliation. After the Civil War, the college gained admission to the Church Institute and the Old Dominion Hospital, but it did not have full authority over them.[13]

Circumstances were similar at the University of Louisville. Proclaiming that from its founding it had been a "practical and demonstrative" institution, the university did not begin to reform its curriculum until the 1890s. Admissions standards continued to be low throughout the 1890s and into the early twentieth century.[14]

Abraham Flexner's 1910 evaluation of conditions at the University of Louisville documented the inadequacy of the laboratory and clinical facilities of the school. Because the university educated so many students—it had an enrollment of 600 in 1910 and was the largest institution of medical education in the country at the time—enormous demands were made on its laboratories and clinics. Flexner found them "inadequate in appointment and teaching force." He was equally critical of the clinical teaching arrangements. Only fifty hospital beds were available to the entire student body, and no regular classes were held in the hospital ward. He ultimately condemned the clinical facilities as "poor in respect to both quality and extent."[15]

Flexner was more pleased by what he found at the College of Physicians and Surgeons in Baltimore than by his discoveries in Richmond and Louisville. He ascertained that, although admissions standards were still very low and some students matriculated without high school diplomas, both clinical and laboratory facilities were more extensive and better maintained in Baltimore than they were in Richmond or Louisville. Although he commented on the weaknesses of the laboratories and blamed them on the payment of faculty royalties, he generally found conditions to be acceptable. He was even more positive about the clinical instruction. The college had control over a 210-bed hospital, conducted regular teaching on the wards, and administered an extensive dispensary.[16] In spite of these propitious comments, however, he ultimately believed that the fate of the institution was sealed as medical education became inextricably linked to university education.[17]

Although these three medical institutions were slow to embrace the reforms initiated at elite medical schools, revision did occur in the late nineteenth and early twentieth centuries. Gradually admissions standards were raised, terms were lengthened, and laboratory and clinical facilities were enhanced. At the University of Louisville, for example, the absorption of the Louisville Medical College, the Hospital College of Medicine, the Kentucky University Medical Department, and the Kentucky School of Medicine helped alleviate some of the overcrowding in the laboratories.[18]

A graded curriculum was introduced at the University of Louisville in 1895, and four years later, the university increased the length of required attendance to four years.[19] In the 1880s, a third, albeit optional, year of lectures was included in the Medical College of Virginia's curriculum. These lectures repeated the previous year's subjects, and it was only in the fall of 1894 that a three-year graded course was approved by the faculty and board of trustees.[20]

Admissions requirements at the Medical College of Virginia were not elevated until the first decade of the twentieth century, when, in 1908, a four-year high school diploma was required. Six years later, at least one year of college was demanded, and in 1916, two years of college became the minimum standard for admission.[21] From a willingness to accept applicants with "a Good English education, including Mathematics and the elementary principles of physics," in 1891 to the requirement of a high school diploma in 1895, the University of Louisville gradually raised its admissions standards through the 1890s.[22]

The difficulties of access to clinical training in Richmond were relieved in 1903 when students at the Medical College of Virginia were given privileges at the newly constructed Memorial Hospital. When the University College of Medicine, a proprietary school founded in 1893, merged with the Medical College of Virginia in 1913, the Medical College of Virginia gained direct control over Memorial Hospital, essentially remedying its clinical deficiencies.

The improvement of medical training at these institutions can also be seen by the increased number of medical students who served as interns, a development that William Rothstein has traced throughout the United States in this era. By his calculations, "the proportion of medical graduates with hospital training grew from an estimated 50 percent in 1904 to 75 percent in 1914."[23] A similar, although slower, rise in the number of internships can also be found among Appalachian graduates of the three institutions under scrutiny.

Of the thirty-four Medical College of Virginia graduates who reported their internship status to the West Virginia State Medical Association between 1900 and 1925, eighteen completed internships. Of those who did undertake internships, 44 percent graduated between 1910 and 1919, and 39 percent graduated between 1920 and 1925. Sixty-eight percent of Medical College of Virginia graduates who received their degrees between 1910 and 1925 completed internships, whereas only 33 percent of those who graduated between 1890 and 1909 pursued internships.[24]

University of Louisville graduates who joined the West Virginia State Medical Association were less likely to have pursued such training than were their colleagues from the Medical College of Virginia. Of the twenty-five graduates who reported their intern status between 1900 and 1925, only twelve had actually completed an internship. Louisville graduates began to pursue internships at an earlier date: 42 percent of those who fulfilled internships graduated be-

Quest for Professional Identity

Table 2.1 Number of Internships Reported by Members of West
Virginia State Medical Association, pre-1890–1925

Decade of Graduation	Interned	Did Not Intern
pre-1890	0	3
1890–99	5	18
1900–1909	25	43
1910–19	38	30
1920–25	24	8
Total	92	102

Source: Membership Records, 1900–1925, West Virginia State Medical
Association Headquarters, Charleston, West Virginia.

tween 1900 and 1909. Internships were not required, however, and
the number of physicians who graduated between 1910 and 1919
and did not complete internships was twice the number of those
who did. Still, however, the popularity of internships as a means
to gain hospital experience increased among graduates in the 1920s.
Three of the four University of Louisville graduates who reported
their internship status between 1920 and 1925 had completed internships.[25]

Of course, not all physicians attended the Medical College of
Virginia or the University of Louisville, but an examination of internships among all West Virginia State Medical Association members
who reported their internship status through 1925 suggests that the
rise in internship opportunities identified by Rothstein may have
come to Appalachian physicians a bit later than it did to other parts
of the country (see table 2.1).

The Medical College of Virginia and the University of Louisville
were less likely to graduate students who interned than were schools
from outside the region whose graduates also practiced in the coalfields.[26] Although regional medical schools were slowly improving
the skills their graduates brought to the mountains, physicians who
were educated at more prestigious and scientifically oriented facilities were already bringing a new level of medical knowledge to the
mountains. Their expertise helped to legitimize the professional
aspirations of less well educated physicians.

All members of the West Virginia State Medical Association who
had graduated from Johns Hopkins University, the University of
Pennsylvania, Harvard University, Vanderbilt University, and Tulane
University who practiced in the West Virginia coalfields reported

pursuing internships. More than three-quarters of those who had graduated from the University of Virginia did so, as did three-quarters of the graduates from George Washington University.[27] Consideration of postgraduate education only confirms that the quality and quantity of knowledge brought to the mountains by those educated outside the region were critical to the creation of medical expertise (see table 2.2). The Universities of Minnesota, Pennsylvania, and Manitoba, as well as Creighton, Loyola, and Tulane Universities and Jefferson Medical College, were all represented by physicians who had completed postgraduate medical training.[28]

Many of the physicians who brought this more advanced medical learning to Appalachia were born outside the region. The arrival of new professionals who possessed more advanced knowledge and who potentially enjoyed extensive connections with regional and national associations helped to shape medicine fundamentally in Appalachia.

An examination of the 192 physicians who provided the West Virginia State Medical Association with information on their birthplaces between 1900 and 1925 reveals that 63 percent were native to the Appalachian states of Virginia, Kentucky, and West Virginia. Of those indigenous to the region, 42 percent possessed postgraduate medical education. One-half of those who relocated to the mountains had postgraduate education. A comparison of the nativity of physicians who did not possess postgraduate medical education with the nativity of those who did indicates that physicians born outside the region were twice as likely to have received postgraduate training as were natives.[29]

As regional medical schools gradually improved their training and outsiders with more prestigious medical diplomas moved to the mountains, physicians closed ranks to foster public recognition of their medical expertise. To do so, doctors formed private medical associations and tied themselves to the state in a crusade to formalize their professional credentials, a process that constitutes Friedson's second pillar of professionalism.[30]

During the early decades of the nineteenth century, northern states had taken the lead in attempting to pass laws defining the parameters of acceptable medical practice. In the Jacksonian era, however, such laws were perceived as unfair constraints on the right of the individual to pursue economic security in the open market and were rejected.[31] Regular physicians reacted to the failure of

Table 2.2 Percentage of Members of West Virginia State Medical
Association Who Attended Graduate School, 1900–1925

School	Graduate School Attendance
Medical College of Virginia	38.0
University of Louisville	41.3
College of Physicians and Surgeons in Baltimore	6.1
University of Virginia	80.0
Johns Hopkins University	50.0
University of Maryland	47.0

Source: Membership Records, 1900–1925, West Virginia State Medical
Association Headquarters, Charleston, West Virginia.

medical licensure by founding the American Medical Association
(AMA) in New York State in 1846. Unable to secure legal validation
of their claim to sole professional legitimacy, they created the AMA to
police medicine through private, professional efforts.[32]

To protect regular doctors' increasingly strident claims to medical
superiority, the AMA denied membership to any physician who did
not enjoy the benefits of an acceptable education or who espoused
an alternative medical philosophy.[33] The creation of an exclusive,
private association with the power to refuse fraternal affiliation to
those who failed to satisfy its criteria became a model for professional development in the United States.[34]

Central Appalachian physicians were both pioneers and late-
comers in the campaign for professionalization. Virginia, for example, possessed a state alliance that predated the AMA. Originally
formed in 1820 by seventeen physicians from Richmond, the Medical Society of Virginia was chartered in 1824 but fell into inactivity
during the 1830s until its revival in 1841. Throughout its early
years, the society was dominated by practitioners from Richmond
and other eastern and coastal cities in the state. Physicians from the
interior and mountain districts agitated against Richmond's control
of the association and insisted that statewide representation be assured. They achieved that goal in 1858, but their success was short-
lived since the society suspended its activities in 1859 and was
moribund until after the Civil War.[35]

Although physicians from Richmond and the Tidewater region
overshadowed the early history of the Medical Society of Virginia,
the revitalization of the association after the Civil War was initiated

by practitioners from the interior and mountain regions of the state. Doctors from Lynchburg and Abingdon played key roles in motivating Virginia's practitioners to reorganize in 1870, and a physician from Lynchburg, Dr. Landon Edwards, served as the first president of the reconstituted society.[36]

Urban physicians also dominated the early history of the Kentucky State Medical Society. Founded in 1851, the society was organized in the chambers of the Kentucky senate in Frankfort, indicating the social and political prestige of its early members. At this first meeting, the physicians adopted the AMA's code of ethics and denied sectarians such as homeopaths or other irregularly trained healers membership.[37]

After statehood separated them from their Virginia brethren in 1863, West Virginia physicians were compelled to create their own state medical association. Formed in Wheeling in 1867, the Medical Society of West Virginia was the last state medical association to be established in the nation at that time. Like their colleagues in Kentucky, West Virginia physicians also adopted the AMA's code of ethics and formally wed themselves to the allopathic, or regular, medical model.[38]

West Virginia physicians were exceptionally vociferous in asserting the sanctity of their profession. According to the booklet they published to celebrate the organization of their society, "The true physician . . . stands upon a lofty eminence, clothed with the authority of science to interpret nature." The pamphlet proclaimed that "no calling represents more fully or more honorably than ours, the intellectual tendency of the times in which we live" and that "a pervading sense of progress is everywhere at work in the medical world."[39]

In spite of their declarations, members of the West Virginia State Medical Association, as it was later renamed, perceived themselves to be vulnerable to challenges by competing healers. Dr. C. H. Maxwell, a physician from the northern West Virginia town of Morgantown, was appalled by the status of his state association when he surveyed it in 1907. Since local associations were lacking in many sections of the state, physicians were thwarted in their attempts to monitor the practice of medicine. He asserted that the inability of West Virginia's physicians to seize control of the definition and regulation of medicine had adverse consequences for the profession as well as for the population of the state. Maxwell warned that West Virginians had not "been trained" and that they had not been "taught" that communicable disease was a "shame." Having failed to "create the proper public sentiment," doctors had not yet fully convinced the public that they alone possessed expertise as healers.[40]

The weakness of medical societies in isolated sections of Appalachia deterred the promotion of such "public sentiment." In 1905, for example, none of the eastern Kentucky counties of Clay, Harlan, Jackson, Knott, Lee, Letcher, Menifee, Perry, and Morgan contained chapters of the Kentucky State Medical Society. Some county societies grew very little over the next few years. No medical association had been established in Menifee County by 1911, and associations in Harlan, Jackson, Knott, Leslie, Owsley, and Perry Counties had enrollments of five or fewer each that year.[41] In southern West Virginia, the McDowell County Medical Society often held joint meetings with colleagues from Mingo and Mercer Counties in an effort to promote professional solidarity and increase the size of the gatherings.[42] As recently as the late 1920s, physicians in southwestern Virginia assembled in conclaves that included physicians from throughout the Virginia mountains as well as from southern West Virginia.[43]

But these conditions began to change as industrialization brought a critical mass of better-educated doctors to the mountains. These physicians, unlike earlier practitioners, were committed to professional development and affiliation. When coal production boomed in Bell County, Kentucky, in the 1900s, the number of new, young physicians increased significantly as the population rose.[44] The Bell County Medical Society, which had only nine members in 1905, grew to include thirty-two physicians by 1911. Harlan, Letcher, Perry, and Pike County medical associations also grew during the development of the Kentucky coalfields in the 1910s and 1920s.[45]

The creation and expansion of local medical associations in Appalachian counties did not ensure full participation or engagement with state medical associations. Unlike their established compatriots in more populated counties, members of mountain medical societies were seldom represented on state committees. Physicians from eastern Kentucky contributed very few articles to the *Kentucky Medical Journal* and often failed even to submit copies of their minutes to the state association, suggesting the often moribund nature of their local chapters.[46]

In part, medical societies were weak because environmental conditions in the mountains discouraged fraternal camaraderie. Champions of county medical associations struggled to entice potential members to travel long distances under difficult circumstances to attend meetings. In 1911, fifteen Floyd County, Kentucky, physicians were eligible to become members of the county medical association; none of them joined, however, essentially terminating the organization's existence that year.[47] Membership in the Knott County Medical Association, which peaked at five in 1910, declined to four in 1911 and sank to a new low of only two in 1914.[48] Dr. Maurice Kaufmann recalled that, even as late as the 1930s, the lengthy trip from his home in Cumberland, Kentucky, to the county seat at Harlan deterred the other Cumberland practitioner from attending medical society meetings there.[49]

State medical associations offered little support to these nascent local societies. Physicians in Raleigh and Mingo Counties in West Virginia received minimal assistance from the state association when they pursued legal action against sectarian healers in their communities. An article in the *West Virginia Medical Journal* questioned whether the state association was even aware of the important work being initiated by its county affiliates in the southern part of the state.[50]

Appalachian county societies may have received minimal assistance and exerted little influence because they brought insignificant income to their state associations. In 1913, the organized medical associations of Letcher, Knott, and Menifee Counties contributed less than $7 each to the state society's coffers. This was substantially less than the amount offered by other county associations.[51]

Weakened by the difficulty of organizing a relatively small number of potential members over rugged terrain, doctors struggled to establish unity within mountain medical communities. Aware of their vulnerability, physicians from the southern coal regions of West Virginia argued that any effort to protect physicians' interests had to be based on consolidated action. "It behooves us," an article in the *West Virginia Medical Journal* claimed, "to double our efforts in the work of organization and have the name of every eligible physician in the State added to the roll of members of the Association."[52] The Wythe County, Virginia, Medical Society expressed similar sentiments as early as 1874.[53]

County medical societies played an important role in the transformation of medical knowledge in Central Appalachia. By allying with other physicians, especially those who were younger and better educated, newly arrived doctors could help create a counterforce to offset the influence of older, established physicians who possessed less scientific training but who often enjoyed the trust of the community. Organized physicians could also use their corporate strength to fight new sectarian opponents and lobby for elevated licensing standards.

Medical societies in Appalachia were, by and large, dominated by younger, degreed physicians. A survey of three southern West Virginia county societies demonstrates that, with few exceptions, organized medicine was shaped by the interests of recently graduated, better-educated physicians. The membership lists of the medical societies of McDowell, Mingo, and Raleigh Counties in 1906 suggest that younger physicians were both the rank and file and the leaders of organized medicine in the mountains. The McDowell County Medical Society, the largest of the alliances under scrutiny, had twenty-two members in 1906. Of those twenty-two, one received his degree in 1872, one in 1887, and the rest between 1890 and 1905. Nine earned their diplomas between 1900 and 1905. The president of the society, Dr. W. L. Johnston, completed his degree at the University College of Medicine in Richmond in 1899. The secretary, Dr. W. E. Cook, graduated from the Medical College of Virginia in 1901; Dr. H. B. Stone, the group's treasurer, completed his medical education at the same institution in 1903.[54]

A similar pattern existed in Mingo County that year: all nine members of the county society earned degrees between 1890 and 1905. Five of the nine graduated between 1900 and 1905. The leadership of the Mingo County Medical Society was equally youthful. Dr. Sherwood Dix, president of the local association, completed his medical degree in 1899 and received his license to practice medicine in West Virginia in 1903. The secretary-treasurer of the Mingo society graduated in 1905.[55]

The Raleigh County Medical Society's president, Dr. W. W. Hume, finished his studies at the University of Virginia in 1901. His first vice president, Dr. A. S. Abshire, was slightly older, having graduated from the College of Physicians and Surgeons in Baltimore in 1891, but Dr. McRae Banks, his second vice president, received his degree from the Medical College of Virginia in 1898. The regular members of the association were equally youthful; in fact, Abshire had earned his degree earlier than anyone else in the organization.[56]

To assure the preeminence of the new medical principles they were learning in the laboratory and clinical sessions that increasingly defined their educations, the young physicians who dominated the medical societies had to denigrate alternative medical philosophies because "the mere existence of competing parties in medicine was a standing rebuke to the claims of orthodoxy to represent a science."[57] Although real challenges to the supremacy of regular medicine disintegrated in the face of the scientific advances of the late nineteenth century, less well educated practitioners, like many of those who practiced in Appalachia, continued to believe themselves vulnerable to sectarian challenges.[58] To strengthen their professional identities and organizations, doctors attacked new sectarian challengers, especially osteopaths and chiropractors, hoping to convince the public that they alone possessed the expert knowledge to diagnose and treat illness.[59]

Physicians argued that sectarians who denied scientific medicine were making an immoral, irresponsible decision. They insisted that adherence to scientific principles was essential to the fulfillment of a doctor's responsibility to protect the community's health. "You know," the secretary of the West Virginia State Medical Association wrote, "that the people are not qualified to select their physician."[60] Because of the public's vulnerability, a doctor from Kentucky stated, educated physicians must assume responsibility for policing medical practice, which included attempting to prevent practitioners who failed to embrace scientific medicine from preying on uninformed citizens.[61] As late as 1930, the Virginia Medical Monthly asserted that the physician "held society together" by protecting it from the dangers of nonscientific medicine.[62]

Younger physicians identified sectarians' rejection of scientific medicine as a hazard to the community, but they also struggled with poorly educated regular doctors whose knowledge of medicine was antiquated and, they believed, potentially dangerous. As younger, more scientifically oriented physicians battled against older doctors rooted in nineteenth-century presumptions, the dramatic differences between the old medicine of the nineteenth century and the developing medicine of the twentieth were revealed. Arguments among physicians over diagnosis and treatment document the tensions between philosophies of practice, but they also reveal that another way in which newly educated physicians sought legitimacy for their medical knowledge was by allying with larger social forces, in this case the state.[63]

Epidemics of smallpox were common throughout eastern Kentucky in the decades around the turn of the century. Like those who faced smallpox outbreaks in more urban settings, Appalachian citizens struggled to make intelligent decisions about their health and well-being while receiving conflicting information from physicians.[64] At times, the divisions were generational, but at other times, physicians who had graduated from medical school in the same year disputed the nature of and appropriate therapy for the illness at hand, illustrating the contested state of medical knowledge in Central Appalachia at the turn of the century. Such tensions demonstrate that, as in the rest of the United States, shifting relationships between doctors and patients and among medical practitioners marked public health developments in this era.[65]

As immunology and pathology improved in the nineteenth century, many well-trained physicians embraced the advantages of vaccination and came to understand the course of smallpox. Older physicians who were not versed in those advances and who defined their therapeutic beliefs in more traditional terms, however, could cause enormous suffering because of their rejection or lack of knowledge of new developments in immunology and bacteriology. Residents of a southern West Virginia community discovered the limitations of nineteenth-century medicine in 1881 when a self-taught physician named Hess mistook smallpox for chickenpox and failed to observe the appropriate precautions. His inability to diagnose and respond to the disease allowed a deadly epidemic to spread through the villages of eastern Mercer and western Pocahontas Counties.[66]

Similar misjudgments took place throughout the Kentucky mountains. At times, older physicians, firmly rooted in the empirical tradition, insisted that their treatments were adequate and confidently resisted efforts by younger physicians to quarantine patients and vaccinate communities. Often allied with their local county court, these older doctors vigorously defended their treatment philosophies, as did some younger physicians who followed in their footsteps and rejected the new revelations of scientific discoveries.[67]

When smallpox broke out in Jackson County, Kentucky, in 1898, the state board of health sent Dr. B. W. Smock, a sanitary inspector from the board's headquarters in Bowling Green, to assess the situation and offer aid to the county court, the agency that oversaw the county board of health. When he arrived, he was assured by Dr. Charles M. Azbill that the residents were only suffering from a "breaking out disease" that was very "ketching." An autopsy on one of the victims, according to Azbill, revealed that he had been "pisened." Azbill, an 1890 graduate of the University of Louisville, staunchly opposed Smock's diagnosis of smallpox and allied with the Jackson County court to resist Smock's efforts to vaccinate and quarantine residents. In response, Smock, under the authority of the state board, reorganized the Jackson County Board of Health and replaced Azbill with Dr. N. M. Clark, an 1891 graduate of the University of Louisville.[68]

Although they had received their educations at the same institution and probably overlapped as classmates, Azbill and Clark held different views of the etiology and treatment of smallpox. By allying with the state, which was expanding its reach into the daily lives of eastern Kentuckians, Clark helped further his ideas of scientific medicine. Because Azbill associated himself with the ultimately antiquated county court system, he was displaced.[69] The accuracy of Smock and Clark's diagnosis and their success in curbing the outbreak constituted a public triumph by the practitioners of scientific medicine in Jackson County.

Public health offices were often staffed by younger physicians and became vehicles for fostering change and introducing medical innovations to Appalachian people.[70] In southern West Virginia in 1908, for example, city boards of health in Beckley, Bluefield, Bramwell, Fayetteville, Matewan, Oak Hill, Princeton, Welch, and Williamson were all manned by physicians who had received degrees in the previous ten years. The same was true at the county boards of health in that region.[71]

Older physicians could display remarkable tenacity in holding onto public health positions. In Dickenson County, Virginia, two of the three doctors on the county board of medicine in 1910 were recent graduates, but one had received his degree thirty years earlier. In Russell County, Dr. W. S. Gilmer, who earned his degree from the Medical College of Virginia in 1869, still occupied a position on the board of health in 1910. In all of the Appalachian counties in Virginia, in fact, at least one older physician continued to sit on the county board of health in the first decade of the twentieth century.[72]

In Kentucky, the shift toward younger, if not always better-educated, physicians began in the 1890s. By 1896, the boards of health of Bell, Breathitt, Harlan, Knox, and Letcher Counties were controlled by physicians who had received their degrees quite recently. In other counties, no young physicians had made their way onto the boards of health. Clay County's board, for example, was administered by men who had graduated in the 1870s. Dr. J. D. Kincaid, who had earned his medical license through a brief medical course and a preceptorship in the 1840s, was the sole health officer in Boyd County.[73]

The persistence of older physicians and the recalcitrance of younger ones who resisted the innovations promised by scientific medicine deterred the professional development so desired by career-minded physicians and revealed the perseverance of older traditions of medical care in which physicians earned as much respect for their community and family ties as for their knowledge.[74] To protect and elevate their medical prestige and help "narrow the range of choice," physicians vigorously pursued medical licensure in order to create a formal credential that recognized their expertise.[75]

State campaigns to regulate medicine were revived after the Civil War.[76] During the middle decades of the nineteenth century, public opinion had demanded that the government protect the free market and the rights of the individual, but fifty years later, the popular will insisted that the government assume a more interventionist role in protecting the citizenry's welfare. This trend was most clearly evidenced in the growing support for public health programs, but it was also revealed by the passage of regulations to establish prerequisites for medical licensing by state legislatures.[77]

The Virginia State Medical Examining Board was founded in 1884. Although it was an official state agency, the first board was composed of men nominated and elected by the Medical Society of Virginia, illustrating the close connections that existed between the state and organized medicine.[78] Established physicians throughout Virginia favored the board's creation, but doctors whose education and professional training had not prepared them to pass an examination written and administered by well-educated physicians expressed strong sentiment against it.[79]

Within the first year of the board's existence, a rural Virginia physician who failed to pass the required examination for licensure challenged the board's right to interfere in the practice of medicine. With the assistance of his father, who was an attorney, Dr. B. B. Halsey questioned the legality of the board's prosecution of physicians who practiced without first receiving a license from the state. Identifying himself as "Clio," the senior Halsey authored a series of letters to the board that mimicked the republican rhetoric of the Revolutionary Era. In these epistles, the author condemned the "tyrannical authority" exhibited by the state as it assumed the right to regulate the practice of medicine. Although his father presented a substantial case, the younger Halsey was prosecuted for practicing medicine without a license and ultimately was found guilty.[80]

Other doctors educated at less renowned schools like the Medical

College of Virginia or trained by a preceptor joined the Halseys in questioning the right of the state to regulate the practice of medicine. Rural physicians who opposed the formation of the board were discomfited by the overrepresentation of urban doctors on the board, particularly those from Richmond.[81] Many ambitious young medical students were also disturbed by the overtly elitist language used by the board to describe its plans to restrict the type of people who practiced medicine. One of the missions of the board, its members determined, was to ensure "that the class of persons who are unfitted by education or capacity to adorn our noble profession will be restrained from entering upon its study."[82]

Students at the Medical College of Virginia in Richmond expressed their concerns about the constraints the board placed on those who sought to practice medicine in an 1886 letter to the board. The students, anxious about their professional and economic futures, wrote: "The sole object of the law regulating the practice of medicine and surgery is a selfish one—i.e. to prevent competition. Medicine is studied and practiced for the sake of profit and gain and not for 'sweet charities sake.' . . . Competition is the right of this as well as of other trades."[83]

The students correctly perceived that the state was attempting to limit competition. By recognizing that educated physicians possessed specialized knowledge, the Virginia State Board of Medicine was beginning the process of extending formal credentials to practitioners who had special expertise based on their education and training. Medical licensing, therefore, was a critical step in the professionalization of medicine.[84]

Like their colleagues in Virginia, Kentucky doctors began to regulate medical practice in the 1880s. The strength of its non-Appalachian membership enabled the Kentucky State Medical Society to exert significant influence over the state government's policies toward medical practice.[85] The association's authority was reinforced by the lengthy careers of Drs. Joseph N. McCormack and Arthur T. McCormack, a father and son duo who served as officers of the medical alliance as well as directors of the state board of health. Their intimate ties with both of these institutions symbolized the intrinsic connections that bound the private medical association to government in the Bluegrass state.[86]

Dr. Joseph McCormack, who eventually played a critical role in the reorganization of the AMA in the early 1900s, pushed the Kentucky government to enact strong public health laws in the 1880s.

He also convinced state legislators that the best way to protect the commonwealth's population was to bring sectarians under the government's oversight as quickly as possible. Therefore, in 1888, the state passed a medical practice law that established standards for sectarians at the same time that it created provisions for the supervision of regular doctors.[87]

Effective laws detailing the requirements for medical licensing helped doctors in Virginia and Kentucky by clearly delineating the criteria for medical practice. In West Virginia, however, explicitly defined standards for medical licensing were more difficult to secure. Without a large, well-educated population of urban practitioners, the physicians' lobby in West Virginia found it difficult to push its initiatives through the state legislature. Originally written in 1881, the state's ordinances overseeing the practice of medicine were revised in 1895 and then again in 1907. As a consequence of the state's ineffective and unclear licensing requirements, sectarians flocked to West Virginia in the late nineteenth and early twentieth centuries.[88]

During the tussle over revising the state's regulations in 1907, osteopaths managed to convince the West Virginia legislature to license them. This, according to one regular doctor, allowed "a new irregular sect to be inflicted on the State." Like osteopaths, chiropractors, referred to in the *West Virginia Medical Journal* as "the latest of the many new frauds . . . to have appeared in this fraud-cursed State," also pursued legal recognition.[89]

In the 1920s, West Virginia physicians, fearful of the new economic and philosophical challenges posed by the growing strength of chiropractors, opposed their licensure by the state.[90] They were particularly unyielding in their refusal to compromise with the chiropractors and were piqued when Governor Howard Gore allowed a bill licensing chiropractors to become a law.[91] Gore and other politicians who supported or at least tolerated the chiropractors' bill were responding to the popularity of alternative medical treatments among their constituents.

Like their West Virginia colleagues, physicians from Virginia had to react to the growing power of chiropractors.[92] During the 1926 legislative session, chiropractors lobbied the Virginia legislature for the establishment of a separate licensing board to oversee their practices. Creating such a body would free them from the control of regular doctors, who dominated the state board of medical examiners, and would allow them to freely practice chiropractic medicine. The Medical Society of Virginia opposed the bill and successfully lobbied for its defeat, although a last-ditch effort by the chiropractors was overcome by only one vote.[93]

Physicians who opposed sectarian medicine vigorously exhorted state governments to enforce medical licensing laws. Local physicians exposed those who, they argued, violated the law by overstepping the proscriptions placed on alternative healers by state governments. Physicians were frustrated in this endeavor, however, by the determination of many Appalachian residents to protect their choices in the medical marketplace.

Appalachian county prosecutors, who were charged with pursuing violators of the medical practice statutes, seldom initiated criminal suits against alternative healers without the direct intervention of the local medical society.[94] In part, their hesitancy grew out of the ambiguity of the laws that governed medical practice.[95] But they were also responding to the wishes of local citizens who patronized and supported the rights of alternative practitioners. When county attorneys did initiate criminal cases against sectarians, residents frequently contested the charges or refused to give evidence against the accused, often actually testifying on behalf of the sectarians. Local juries sometimes refused to return bills of indictment against sectarians in spite of the often overwhelming testimony given against them.[96]

In 1924, just one year before the chiropractor law was passed, the West Virginia State Medical Association issued an appeal to its members to pursue local cases against sectarians, especially chiropractors. The association was particularly frustrated by its component societies' inability to successfully persecute sectarians. The Raleigh County Medical Society, for example, won a rare judgment against a chiropractor, but the convicted practitioner appealed the decision and took his case to the state supreme court. According to the state association, Mingo was the only other county that had succeeded in securing an indictment against a chiropractor. In that case, however, the jury returned a verdict of not guilty in three minutes.[97]

Other West Virginians shared the approval of sectarian care expressed by the Mingo County jury. As regular doctors fought against them during the 1925 legislative session, chiropractors persuaded their supporters to sign a petition calling for passage of a licensing bill for chiropractors. Before the legislative battle was over, advocates of the chiropractic method had gained more than 7,000 signatures on their petition.[98]

Physicians saw their fight against sectarian healers as an extension of their moral responsibility to protect the community from practitioners who rejected the advances of scientific medicine. But in many cases, the public did not want to be protected, preferring free choice in the medical marketplace over limitations imposed by regular physicians. Apparently convinced that their responsibilities to the public included controlling sectarian healers, doctors ignored public sentiment and attempted to ally with the government to impose their own expectations about the practice of medicine on the community.

Legal restrictions that limited the actions of competing professionals, however, often had few consequences for the daily lives of rural Appalachian people. Such laws might give one provider advantages over another, but laws passed in Frankfort, Richmond, or Charleston could not immediately reshape the expectations of country people. The gradually improving medical curriculum and the benediction bestowed by the acquisition of a formal medical license were not enough to undermine centuries-old traditions in the mountains. The persistence of midwifery in Appalachia illustrates the failure of educational improvement and state licensing to eliminate competing healers as well as the inability of educated physicians to interject themselves into gender-specific private spaces.

Among Appalachian women, midwifery followed the pattern Charlotte Borst found among "neighbor-women" in rural Wisconsin. Lacking formal medical education, many Appalachian midwives delivered only a few babies, and their assistance was part of a familial or community network of reciprocity.[99] Although a few midwives delivered a significantly higher number of infants than these "neighbor-women" delivered, they did not possess extensive formal education and clearly failed to meet even the most generous standard of professional development.[100]

Birth records in Logan and Mingo Counties in southern West Virginia give some indication of the world in which lay midwives practiced just before the turn of the twentieth century. These two counties, which were united until Mingo was separated from Logan in 1895, sit squarely in the middle of the Appalachian coalfields and are best known as the site of some of the region's most violent labor conflicts.[101] Lying just across the Tug River from Kentucky, these were the hills where the Hatfields and McCoys acted as foot soldiers in a complicated battle over the shape of commercial and industrial development.[102]

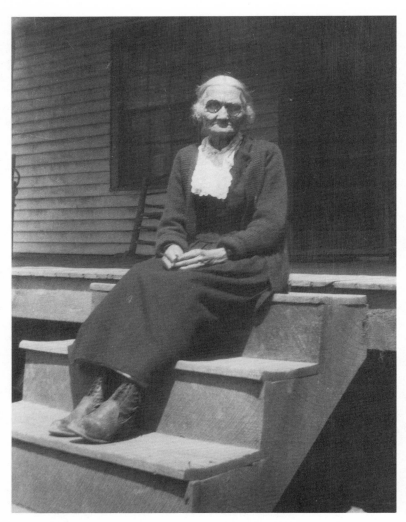

Appalachian doctors struggled to displace midwives like this elderly woman from eastern Kentucky during the first decades of the twentieth century. Audio-Visual Archives, Special Collections and Archives, University of Kentucky Libraries.

The lives of lay midwives, the women they aided, and the doctors they competed against and sometimes cooperated with seem to reflect little of the tension that produced such bloody events. In a different way, however, the campaign by physicians to replace lay midwives was another example of the creeping processes of industrialization and modernity in Appalachia.

Although most existent birth records in Central Appalachia from

Table 2.3 Percentage of Reported Deliveries by Midwives, Logan County, West Virginia, 1890–1900

Year	Deliveries by Midwives
1890	56
1891	47
1892	29
1893	43
1894	44
1895	35
1896	27
1897	41
1898	44
1899	45
1900	40

Source: *Logan County Births,* 1872–1900, 1–52.

this era do not indicate the names of birth attendants, Logan County records from 1889 through 1900 do. From these records, it is possible to trace the movement of physicians into the birthing rooms of Central Appalachia as well as to acquire some knowledge of the women who delivered many of the babies born in the county.

As table 2.3 indicates, lay midwives delivered a significant number of babies in Logan County in the 1890s. An examination of the locations of births in the county reveals the importance of midwives in rural districts, suggesting a clear division between countryside and town and between agricultural and mining communities. Infants born in towns, especially in the county seat of Logan, were typically delivered by physicians. Women who gave birth in coal camps were also usually attended by physicians. In rural communities where agriculture and timbering still dominated, however, midwives continued to care for significant numbers of women.[103]

Logan County records do not consistently document the location of births outside the coal camps or the county seat of Logan, but some patterns that do emerge indicate that, like rural Wisconsin midwives, Appalachian midwives practiced in a small geographical area.[104] Table 2.4 shows the percentages of babies delivered by the most active Logan County midwives from 1890 through 1900. Susan White, for example, delivered all of the infants who were born in her neighborhood along Mill Creek in this ten-year period. She was also the only person who reported delivering babies in

Table 2.4 Percentage of Reported Deliveries by Most Active
Midwives, Logan County, West Virginia, 1890–1900

Midwife	Deliveries by Midwives	Total Deliveries
Susan Berkeley	7.9	3.2
Dorcas Dempsey	10.0	4.0
Malinda Ellis	15.0	6.1
Penelope Thompson	10.0	4.0
Isabel White	22.4	9.2
Susan White	6.6	2.7

Source: *Logan County Births*, 1872–1900, 1–52.

Hewitt. Malinda Ellis seemed to be the midwife of choice among
women who gave birth in the Sand Lick area, and Penelope Thompson appeared to have a monopoly on delivering babies in the
Crawley Creek region.[105]

White, Ellis, and Thompson were among a small group of
women who engaged in extensive midwifery practices; many other
women simply assisted neighbors or relatives and were recorded in
birth records on only one or two occasions each. Of twenty-seven
women who reported their attendance at births, fourteen had assisted in only one or two deliveries each; the vast majority of those
women, twelve of fourteen, were present for only one birth. On the
other hand, White, Ellis, Thompson, and three other women had
assisted at twenty-five or more births each and, combined, had
delivered 77 percent of the infants born under the care of midwives.[106]

Table 2.5 gives the number of births per year by the most active
Logan County midwives. These numbers reveal that, although midwives were being challenged by the arrival of new physicians, they
were not being displaced by them since younger midwives were
stepping in as older women withdrew from practice due to old age,
ill health, or death.

With the exception of Isabel White, no midwife worked consistently throughout the decade. Midwives' practices were relatively
brief because, as historians of midwifery have illustrated, midwifery
was essentially an art that women fit around their domestic obligations. As their children grew up and began to take care of themselves, these married women could commit more of their time to
their craft. When they became elderly, they were less able, or perhaps less willing, to wait for the completion of a potentially lengthy

Table 2.5 Number of Deliveries by Most Active Midwives, Logan County, West Virginia, 1890–1900

Midwife	1890	1891	1892	1893	1894	1895	1896	1897	1898	1899	1900
Susan Berkeley	2	0	0	13	12	3	0	0	0	0	0
Dorcas Dempsey	10	11	3	8	6	0	0	0	0	0	0
Malinda Ellis	0	0	0	0	0	8	10	9	10	12	8
Penelope Thompson	0	0	0	0	0	0	0	9	8	12	9
Isabel White	6	17	3	11	7	4	5	11	8	6	6
Susan White	5	15	3	2	0	0	0	0	0	0	0

Source: *Logan County Births, 1872–1900,* 1–52.

labor. Older women had the freedom to step out of midwifery because other younger women were approaching the point in their life cycles at which they could take up the burden.[107]

Four of the six midwives named in tables 2.4 and 2.5 were listed in either the 1880 or 1900 manuscript census for Logan or Mingo County. The census data indicates that in 1890 Penelope Thompson was forty-seven, Malinda Ellis was fifty, Susan White was fifty-nine, and Dorcas Dempsey was seventy-six. As would be expected, Thompson and Ellis were just beginning their midwifery practices as White and Dempsey were ending theirs.[108]

When Thompson began her practice in 1897, her youngest child was twenty-one years old. Having raised six children, she possessed the basic knowledge and personal experience of childbirth required of a midwife. Like Thompson, Dorcas Dempsey and White, as well as Charlotte Burgess and Barbara Dempsey, midwives who delivered more than ten babies in the 1890s, all earned their legitimacy through the birth of their own children.[109]

All of these women also enjoyed the authority that came with marriage and economic stability. With the exception of Ellis, who was a widow, all were married to farmers who claimed ownership of their land. Their families also represented stability in a rapidly growing region. Burgess, Barbara Dempsey, Dorcas Dempsey, Thompson, and White, as well as their husbands, were all born in

West Virginia. They indicated to the census taker that their parents were also West Virginia natives.[110] Their statements indicate their local identities rather than state allegiance since West Virginia did not exist when they or their parents were born.

As longtime residents of the area, these women and their families experienced the industrial transformation firsthand. One of the Dempsey clan, for example, was a fatality of the Hatfield-McCoy feud in 1888.[111] For most of these women, the transition to modern industrial life was not so violent, but the arrival of new physicians seeking to provide care to women who traditionally had looked to midwives challenged established norms.

By 1886, four physicians were practicing in Logan County.[112] That number had increased to six in 1896, although Mingo County had been separated from Logan by that time.[113] These physicians immediately began to displace midwives in the town of Logan and in the coal camps. In these communities, physicians became the established childbirth attendants, quickly making significant inroads into the market. Table 2.6 shows the percentage of births by five physicians in Logan County from 1890 through 1900.

Like midwives, physicians who practiced longer delivered more babies, but the younger age at which physicians began their careers meant that they could pursue them longer. Unlike midwives, physicians did not have to fit their childbirthing duties around their domestic lives or delay their entry into the field until their parental obligations were fulfilled. S. B. Lawson, who graduated from the Baltimore Medical College in 1894 as a young man, was still practicing in Logan County in 1917. M. H. Waldron, who practiced in the part of Logan County that became Mingo, came to the region after earning his degree at an eclectic college in Ohio in 1867. In 1917, he was still practicing in Mingo County.[114]

The speed with which these physicians began to challenge midwives indicates that some women readily embraced the possibility of having a male birth attendant. On the other hand, however, midwives continued to hold their own in many sections of the county. As table 2.3 indicates, midwifery certainly declined in the 1890s, but it did not vanish, and it could be argued that a 16 percent drop over a ten-year period in which new competitors were entering the field might be seen as relatively successful resistance to change.

In part, midwives maintained their standing because they had so much in common with native residents. As noted above, educated physicians often came from established families with extensive ties

Table 2.6 Percentage of Reported Deliveries by Named Physicians, Logan County, West Virginia, 1890–1900

Physician	Deliveries by Physicians	Total Deliveries
M. F. French	35.0	20.7
W. H. Pardue	16.0	9.4
S. B. Lawson	20.0	11.6
H. H. Bryan	4.6	2.3
G. E. Bryan	4.2	2.5

Source: *Logan County Births, 1872–1900, 1–52.*

to institutions outside the region.[115] Midwives, on the other hand, tended to be from more rural agricultural families and to find their client base among those who shared their background. Although nothing as strong as ethnicity held midwives and their patients together, a bond based on shared experience as rural neighbors certainly united them.[116]

The coal camp, on the other hand, was a new social space in which the physicians could displace midwives. The newly arrived residents of these recently constructed villages were often isolated from their social and familial ties, which provided educated physicians with a unique opportunity to promote, and even impose, their practices on the inhabitants.[117] Their success in this endeavor is demonstrated by the low number of deliveries overseen by midwives in the coal counties of West Virginia during the 1920s and 1930s. In the mining camps of Raleigh County, an investigator for the Children's Bureau reported in 1923, 97 percent of the deliveries had been assisted by physicians.[118] At the same time, midwives attended a significant percentage of deliveries in less industrialized, sparsely settled counties such as Webster and Clay. Residents of urban communities and mining counties such as Fayette, McDowell, and Mercer, however, relied almost exclusively on physicians to deliver their infants, a consequence of the dependency on company doctors that developed with the arrival of outside corporations.[119]

Coal camp doctors brought the message of physician-assisted childbirth to the industrial workforce of Central Appalachia, but physicians also looked to the state to aid them by regulating or even eliminating lay midwives. In West Virginia, a 1925 law regulating midwifery obligated midwives to register with the county court or health department. Faced with the demand that they pay a licensing fee and recognize the state's right to oversee midwifery, some women simply refused to submit to the government's commands. Minnie Hammonds, who assisted parturient women in the hills of central West Virginia, rejected the local doctor's insistence that she acquire a license. Although her relationship with that physician remained generally cordial, she resisted the state's demands, ignoring the government's requirements and satisfying her own objectives instead.[120]

Technically outside the letter of the law, Hammonds continued her practice, providing rural, often poor, women with access to what Judith Barrett Litoff has described as the lower level of childbirth assistance.[121] Her services were not recognized by the West Virginia government, but she played a critical role in her community, aiding those who could not secure care from a physician.[122]

The failure of legislation to eliminate lay midwifery in eastern Kentucky was exhibited by the continued reliance of Appalachian women on their traditional birth attendants. A report compiled by Annie Veech, a female physician who directed Kentucky's Bureau of Maternal and Child Health, documented the activity of lay midwives in three counties of that state in 1922. In that year, 2,500 midwives delivered 18 percent of the infants born in Kentucky. In Appalachian Kentucky, however, they remained the principal birth attendants. Leslie County was the home of one physician and forty-three midwives. He delivered 13 percent of the county's infants, and the midwives delivered 87 percent. The five physicians who practiced in Knott County delivered nearly 9 percent of the infants born in 1922, and the fifty-five midwives who worked there assisted at the births of 91 percent. Of the 229 babies born in Owsley County, three physicians delivered 29 percent, and fifty-three midwives delivered 71 percent.[123]

The persistence of lay midwifery was rooted in a shifting combination of rurality, distance from educated healers, and poverty. But it was also motivated by the tradition of community-based healers that had shaped rural life since European settlement in the mountains. In her dissertation on lay midwifery in Appalachian North Carolina, Cathy Melvin Efird describes the traditional midwife: "The southern granny midwife of the early twentieth century, then, was basically like other people in her community. She lived a simple agrarian life punctuated by her attendance at the birth of her neighbors' and kinfolks' children. She was a member of the community first and a health practitioner second. She was a non-professional who relied on natural remedies and who practiced in response to a spiritual call. These characteristics indicate that the granny midwife role was firmly entrenched in the traditional medical system."[124]

Midwives and other lay and folk healers primarily identified themselves as members of their families and communities. They possessed recognized skills that they were obligated, as members of the community, to share with others in exchange for whatever patients might have to offer. Physicians, who were wedded to a scientifically focused professional model, rejected both the treatment policies of traditional healers and the social customs and expectations that sustained them. Since traditional attendants were not professionally ambitious, however, physicians were confounded as to how to thwart their practice. Legislative campaigns had some effect, but they were less successful against folk healers than against sectarians. The practice of traditional health care did not rely on professional or even legal standing. Some midwives chose to apply for licensing in order to improve the quality of their practice, not because of the state's requirements. Others simply ignored the laws, continuing their practice but avoiding the state's prohibitions by refusing to accept money for their services.[125]

Having consolidated a body of knowledge that could be defined as expertise, regular physicians struggled to ensure public recognition of their specialized skills. As members of private medical associations and local boards of health, physicians campaigned for public acceptance of the new medical principles they advocated. By crusading for state licensing laws that limited the autonomy of sectarians, regular doctors affirmed their ability to define acceptable medical knowledge and practice, exhibiting their success at fulfilling Friedson's second requirement for professionalization.[126]

That achievement, however, meant relatively little if potential patients failed to embrace doctors' new expertise or to obey laws proscribing the practices of sectarians or traditional healers. Many mountain residents were unprepared or unwilling to make the epistemological shift necessary to embrace scientific medicine at the beginning of the twentieth century. As an impoverished people, nineteenth-century Appalachian residents had relatively few contacts with educated physicians; their bombardment by newly arrived doctors fundamentally redefined their access to scientific medicine, but it could not immediately shake their traditional reliance on lay healers and midwives. To change those beliefs, physicians had to change Appalachian culture, especially the presumptions women held about labor and delivery. Fortuitously for them, their determination to do so coincided with a growing expression of maternalist concern among middle-class women across the United States.

Quest for Professional Identity

What the

Women's Clubs

Can Do

Physicians looked beyond their internal vehicles and sought external alliances in order to enhance the social as well as the professional prestige of their occupation. They continued to rely on the state to regulate competing healers and to use their private medical associations to promote professionalization, but they sought nonprofessional allies to assist them in recasting public expectations about health and healing.

By seeking to secure class and social support for their campaign to further the position of scientific medicine, physicians were acknowledging that increasing their professional status required the alteration of contemporary Appalachian society. Whether they inhabited rural mountain communities or bustling mining towns, nonprofessional Appalachians had to be convinced that they were dependent on educated physicians for quality care and healing. Doctors, by themselves, could not impose this new paradigm on residents. Unlike coal operators and timber interests, medical practitioners could not simply purchase land or mineral rights and then, with the tacit support of the state, engage in their chosen economic endeavor at will; instead, they needed the cooperation of clients who would seek out scientific practitioners and agree to compensate them for the care these new patients now believed they needed.

Physicians were fortunate that they initiated their campaign during the same era in which middle-class and affluent women, often newcomers to Appalachia, were casting about for meaningful opportunities to contribute to the developing communities they inhabited or to serve mountain residents they identified as in need of relief. As members of a new middle class that was struggling to reshape the Appalachian landscape to suit its expectations and desires, female volunteers seized the opportunity to promote improved medical care as a way to foster their emerging class standing. At the same time, they engaged in volunteer activities that confirmed their claim to protect the family and the community by reflecting their maternalist ideals. Educated, often affluent, settlement workers, who enjoyed greater freedom from the everyday burdens of home and hearth, joined the crusade to improve the lives of the mountaineers they deemed uniquely worthy of relief; at the same time, their alliance with the physicians furthered their own ambitions. Both groups of women, limited in their ability to acquire social and professional standing on their own, sought to gain legitimacy for their reform efforts by assisting physicians.

Defined by their maternalist identities and beliefs, clubwomen focused their reform activity on improving education, advancing public health efforts, and reducing infant and maternal mortality.[1] Whether condemning poor women as inadequate mothers or identifying them as unfortunate victims, Appalachian clubwomen targeted mothers and children specifically for relief and promoted scientific advances in medicine and child care that were gaining popularity among the middle class across the nation.[2] As the population most likely to have embraced doctors as birth attendants, the middle-class women who made up the club movement were enthusiastic about the intervention of physicians and campaigned to extend the promises doctors offered to other mothers and children.[3] They championed this cause by initiating charitable programs and supporting public information campaigns, adopting tactics used in crusades for municipal housekeeping, mothers' pensions, and protective labor legislation across the nation.[4]

Female reformers forged critical ties with male doctors, but the connections they developed with one another also defined the shape of Progressive Era reform in the Appalachian Mountains. Clubwomen and settlement workers addressed different populations, but they shared similar presumptions about the ideology that legitimized their activism. Guided by maternalist beliefs in their sacred obligation to protect women and children, clubwomen directed their efforts toward meeting the needs of working families in mining camps, whereas settlement workers focused on securing educated practitioners for isolated mountain communities. The two groups targeted different audiences, but middle-class female volunteers frequently provided financial and moral support for settlement

What the Women's Clubs Can Do

projects in rural communities, offering their assistance in the work of the region's better-known reform elite.[5]

Much has been written about the settlement aristocracy, but a great deal less is known about the identities and activities of the middle-class women who labored in their own towns and villages and provided financial resources for settlement programs. Newcomers in rapidly expanding communities, they sought the legitimacy that membership in voluntary benevolent organizations offered.[6] Just as the commercial revolution, as Nancy Hewitt has demonstrated, remade the lives of women in Rochester, New York, years earlier, Appalachian women who were coming to occupy positions in the new middle class used their benevolence work to formalize their station.[7] Inhabiting the same new social space but lacking a "local history," Appalachian clubwomen had to construct a new corporate identity. By examining their experiences, we can begin to see beyond the "dominant theoretical perspectives in regional historiography [that] have tended to render women marginal" and recognize the agency of middle-class women who played a role in shaping the transformation of medical care and Appalachian life in this critical period of the region's history.[8]

Appalachian clubwomen must be seen as local actors in a national movement. Their activities were defined by the region in which they lived, but their ambitions reflected trends shaped by the actions of the national association with which they were affiliated. Accounts of the history of women's voluntary organizations in the twentieth century often begin with the founding of the General Federation of Women's Clubs (GFWC) in the 1890s. A national association of affiliated clubs espousing a myriad of ambitions, the GFWC demanded civic reform and made the concept of municipal housekeeping a common topic of discussion.[9] The creation of the GFWC culminated a century of voluntary benevolent organizing by American women, and its formation represented the achievement of a new level of maturity as well as the nationalization of the movement.[10]

The GFWC had its immediate origins in the voluntary associations of New England and New York. Other clubs had expressed interest in forming a national cooperative association, but it was Sorosis, a league of New York women, that gave birth to the GFWC by inviting representatives from many of the nation's female voluntary organizations to attend an assembly in 1890 celebrating its twenty-first birthday. The GFWC quickly became the nation's most influential association of women volunteers.[11]

The GFWC was, from its earliest beginnings, a moderate, even conservative, association. Local clubs enjoyed significant autonomy in choosing projects, but the national association set the agenda by establishing policy and offering philosophical guidance. The GFWC's leadership demonstrated its conservatism at the 1912 national convention when it rejected a motion from the floor supporting women's suffrage. The association's president "ruled the resolution out of order as not germane to the program of the organization." The GFWC debated the question for two more years before finally agreeing to support the proposal.[12]

During the early years of the GFWC, few southern women took an active role at the national level. Of the fifty-one clubs that signed the federation's charter in 1890, only two, composed of women in New Orleans and in Knoxville, represented states south of the Mason-Dixon line. The official charter granted to the GFWC in 1901 by the U.S. Congress demonstrates the continuation of that pattern: only two of the more than sixty women who signed the charter were from southern states.[13]

Although they were not potent forces in the early years of the GFWC, women from the South and from Central Appalachia did form state federations and associate with the national body soon after its founding. Anne Firor Scott has argued that voluntary organizations actually created important opportunities for southern women, who were bound by a culture that extolled their domestic skills while denying them public autonomy. Southern women, she writes, "had to follow a more devious road to emancipation." Voluntary associations, especially those affiliated with the essentially conservative GFWC, provided an appropriate vehicle for southern females who sought to exert their will in the public domain.[14]

Kentucky was the first southern state to respond to the call for organization and federation. Guided by women from the affluent Bluegrass region who formed the eighteen charter clubs of the Kentucky Federation of Women's Clubs, Kentucky became the fifth state to ally with the GFWC, joining in July 1894. The state association grew quickly, and the GFWC accepted its invitation to hold the 1896 national convention in Louisville.[15]

Women from the Bluegrass and western portions of Kentucky were quite enthusiastic about forming alliances with the state federation; however, the call for organization was either ignored or unheard by women from the eastern mountains. By 1898, the state federation had grown beyond the exclusively Bluegrass contingent

What the Women's Clubs Can Do

that had originally composed its membership, but few clubs existed in the Appalachian region of the state. Clubs from Harrodsburg and Middlesboro had affiliated with the state federation by 1898, but they were dramatically outnumbered by women from the Lexington area and the western river towns.[16] The GFWC archive in Washington, D.C., possesses few records of clubs in the Appalachian region of the state that were active early in the twentieth century.[17] Like scientific medical associations, women's clubs did not immediately take root in the mountains and coal camps of eastern Kentucky.

West Virginia, which lacked the social and financial affluence of central and western Kentucky, did not affiliate with the GFWC for several years after the organization's founding, finally forming a relationship with the national body in 1904. As in Kentucky, the primary initiative for federation came from the more established communities of the state; Wheeling and Charleston, for example, were heavily represented in the early membership of the association.[18]

West Virginia clubwomen described their state as an unsophisticated, rural place with little tradition of voluntary association or organization. Distinct regional divisions split the state. Whereas inhabitants of cities were quick to establish clubs and promote affiliation with the GFWC, rural women in the state's southern mountains were initially much less willing or able to invest their time in such activities. In the first year of the state federation, only one state officer represented a club outside the metropolitan centers.[19] The state did not hold a convention in the southern mountains until 1920, when it met in Bluefield, and did not elect its first southern president until 1927.[20]

Although Virginia enjoyed an extensive network of independent women's social organizations, clubwomen delayed allying themselves with the GFWC as a demonstration of the Old Dominion's continued resistance to any form of racial progressivism.[21] Like their sisters in the Deep South, Virginia's clubwomen refused to join any organization that accepted African Americans on an equal basis with whites.[22] Since several northern states, such as Massachusetts, permitted local clubs to establish their own racial standards for membership, the clubwomen of Virginia rejected an invitation from the GFWC to join the national association. At its 1908 convention in Radford, the state federation demanded that the by-laws of the national federation be changed to expressly deny membership to African American women as a prerequisite to Virginia's affiliation.[23] Having been assured by the national federation of the racial purity of the association, the Virginia federation finally agreed to ally itself with the GFWC in 1910.[24]

Unlike the Appalachian portions of Kentucky and West Virginia, the mountains of Virginia were home to a number of clubs that federated in the early days of the state association. The TAM Club of Christiansburg was one of the charter members of the Virginia Federation of Women's Clubs.[25] By 1915, clubs existed in towns across the mountains of southwestern Virginia; Emory, Tazewell, Blacksburg, Big Stone Gap, Pulaski, and Abingdon all enjoyed the presence of a federated women's club by that time.[26] Clubs in this region were less stable, however, than were their affiliates in more eastern reaches of the state. Both the TAM Club of Christiansburg and the Women's Club of Blacksburg disbanded in the 1910s, the only two clubs in the state federation to falter.[27]

The women who built the Appalachian club movement, like physicians who transformed medicine in the region, represented both the preindustrial agricultural elite and newly arrived outsiders. Married to men who were both native and foreign to the region, these women enjoyed varying degrees of familiarity with the towns and camps in which they lived as well as with the developing middle class with which they came to identify. To solidify their position, they worked to create a corporate identity built on their families' position in the maturing extractive economy and the commercial activity that grew up around it.[28]

Many of the southern West Virginia women who joined clubs in the first decades of the twentieth century were from families established in the region before the expansion of the coal economy. As members of families who made the transition from agriculture and small-scale production to participation in the industrial economy, these women were, as Jane Becker has written, "suspend[ed] between very different worlds."[29] Their families, in some cases, had lived in the region for decades and faced the turmoil created by industrial intrusion, but their experiences demonstrate that some Appalachian families preserved their position during the region's transformation and sometimes even managed to improve it.

When Ella Love married Thomas E. Bibb in Fayette County in 1888, they joined two established families that had increased their status and economic stability through a combination of farming, timbering, and employment as schoolteachers. Both of their fathers were educators, Thomas's father having served as superintendent of the Fayette County schools for sixteen years. As the region's com-

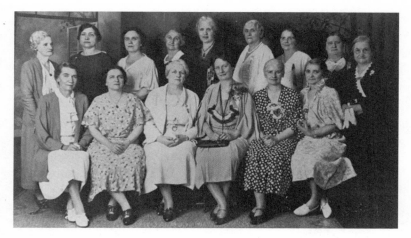

The officers of the Southern District of the West Virginia Federation of Women's Clubs represented the region's increasingly powerful middle class. West Virginia and Regional History Collection, West Virginia University.

mercial economy grew, the Bibbs relocated to Bluefield, where they established a furniture wholesale business that sold wares to residents of mining camps who purchased goods they would have previously made themselves or ordered through catalogs.[30] As the wife of a successful merchant, Ella Love Bibb had made the transformation from country girl to city wife; she joined the Bluefield Women's Club and saw her daughter married to the son of a local politician.[31]

Sallie Holyrod, born in Mercer County in the 1870s, was the daughter of an English woolen manufacturer who came to southern West Virginia as a missionary for the Methodist Episcopal Church in the 1860s. Her brother James taught at Concord State Normal School and was superintendent of schools, and Samuel, another brother, was a physician who served as president of the West Virginia State Medical Association. In 1891, she married William H. McGinnis, a native of Raleigh County whose family had large landholdings rich in coal deposits. McGinnis took advantage of his extensive family ties among the mercantile and legal elite of the district by becoming an attorney representing coal companies and other corporate interests. He served as a state senator and bank director. Sallie Holyrod McGinnis was an officer in the Bluefield Women's Club, and her children continued the family's legal tradition by either becoming lawyers or marrying them.[32]

Like Thomas Bibb, H. H. Ball was a merchant; Ball established the

Hub Clothing Company in Princeton, West Virginia. His wife, Eva Bolin Ball, was a native of Athens, also in Mercer County. The Ball and Bolin families were not as attached to the commercial and legal elite as were the Bibb and McGinnis families, but their experience demonstrates how less well positioned families improved their status during the region's transformation. The Balls were saddlers and harness makers as well as farmers in Russell County, Virginia, in the late nineteenth century. H. H. Ball worked as a timekeeper on the railroad and a manager in several company stores in the coalfields to secure the capital to start his own business. With $1,000 in savings and the aid of friends, he opened his store in the 1910s. By 1921, he was president of the Princeton Business Men's Club and had extended his interests into real estate development. Eva Bolin Ball was an active clubwoman, serving as president of the Princeton Women's Club from 1917 to 1918.[33]

These stories illustrate the transformation of families from a reliance on agriculture to engagement in commercial or professional activity, but we can gain a richer image of the women who joined the clubs by remembering that these local women allied with newly arrived outsiders to form their organizations. This interaction fused a new identity that enabled outsiders as well as locals to reformulate their understanding of themselves as members of the developing Appalachian middle class.

Arabella Rigby Borden, a native of Ohio, came to Bluefield with her husband Chapman. Born in Blacksburg, Virginia, Chapman Borden's father quarried stone for use in the construction of the railroad through that region and became the first postmaster in his area, a position he shared with his son by making him assistant postmaster. When his family's political fortunes changed and his father lost the post office appointment, Chapman Borden worked for the Norfolk and Western Railroad, in turn, as a hotel steward, construction worker, clerk, bookkeeper, and timekeeper. Gradually rising through the ranks at the railroad, he became a facilities manager in Bluefield. That position earned him a seat on the Bluefield Chamber of Commerce as well as membership in the Bluefield Country Club and the Rotary Club. His wife joined the Bluefield Women's Club.[34]

Joe Smith grew up in Raleigh County, West Virginia, the son of farmers. He began work as a printer's devil at fourteen to cover his school expenses. Smith eventually purchased the Raleigh County newspaper but sold it to buy interest in the Beckley National Bank, after which he made himself its president. He was the first mayor of Beckley, served on the city council, was elected to the state senate, and joined the chamber of commerce, the Kiwanis, and the Masons. At thirty-four, he married Christine Carlson, a native of Annapolis, Maryland, who joined the Beckley Women's Club as soon as she arrived in town and, even after giving birth to two sons in rapid succession, remained active in the organization.[35]

Bertha Hamer MacTaggart knew what to expect when she arrived in the coalfields of West Virginia in 1899 since her parents had owned coal mines in Pennsylvania. She married William MacTaggart in Jeansville, Pennsylvania, in 1896. MacTaggart was a Scot whose father had worked as a mine accountant at home but went underground when the family emigrated to Pennsylvania in 1870. The elder MacTaggart was killed in a mining accident in 1881. William, who had begun working with his father as a slate picker when he was eight, supported the family as a miner after his father's death, gradually rising to the position of mine superintendent in Pennsylvania. He attended two years of college at Grove City College in western Pennsylvania and then completed his engineering training through an apprenticeship. As a mining engineer, he worked for the Lehigh Valley Coal Company in Hazelton, Pennsylvania, then the Fairmont Coal Company, before relocating to southern West Virginia to serve as superintendent at the Beaver Coal Company in 1903. His wife was an active member of the Beckley Women's Club, and MacTaggart was a Kiwanian and president of the Beckley Club and was largely responsible for persuading the Beaver Coal Company to donate land for the construction of a community hospital.[36]

Close scrutiny of the Women's Club of Bluefield, West Virginia, as a corporate entity reveals information about the composition of women's clubs and their place in the local community. Founded in 1912 and federated with both the state and national associations a year later, the Bluefield Women's Club was one of the most successful and active clubs in southern West Virginia.[37] By the middle of the 1920s, the club, whose membership averaged around seventy, had become a potent social force in the community.[38] The Bluefield Women's Club produced the first president of the West Virginia Federation of Women's Clubs from the southern mountains when Bethea Brouse Black, the wife of a local dentist, was elected to that position in 1927.[39]

Comparing the club's lists of officers with the city directories offers a partial portrait of the women who were active members of voluntary organizations of this type in the Appalachian Mountains during the early decades of the century. The thirty-three women who can be traced from 1919 through 1932 demonstrate remarkable stability and permanence. Changes in residence by these women and their families were rare, but if the women did relocate, they tended to leave town. Only two of the thirty-three clubwomen listed in the 1919 city directory had moved from one local address to another by 1932. Three other members had apparently left Bluefield since neither they nor their husbands were still listed in the directory.[40]

A majority of the Bluefield officers were married women; only two entries failed to include information on the woman's husband. According to the data provided by the city directories, the composition of the membership of the Bluefield Women's Club would support the claim that clubwomen generally developed their benevolence skills in middle-class homes since the husbands of most of the clubwomen were skilled workers or professionals.[41] The wife of the editor of the local newspaper was a clubwoman, as were the wives of several lawyers, coal operators, dentists, a state supreme court judge, and the local prosecuting attorney. Along with these prestigious professionals, clubwomen were also married to store managers, draftsmen, railroad engineers, and salesmen.[42]

At least three of Bluefield's long-serving clubwomen were married to physicians. Through their marriages, these women volunteers acquired unique insight into the professional objectives of the scientific medical community. Lucille Price's experience exemplified the intimate ties that connected some health advocates and medical practitioners. As the wife of Dr. Samuel W. Price, a prominent physician from Scarbro, West Virginia, who served as the contract doctor for several large coal companies and was appointed to the state board of public health, Lucille Price was thoroughly exposed to medical matters. Price served as an officer in her local women's club and often initiated and managed club-sponsored clinics. She was also involved in the antituberculosis campaign, serving as an officer at both the state and the national levels.[43] In addition to these personal accomplishments, she was elected to a seat in the West Virginia House of Delegates, where she made public health concerns a central focus of her legislative efforts.[44]

Other less prominent women enjoyed significant relationships with men in the medical community. Gazelle Hundley Hume, the state chair of the Public Health Committee of the West Virginia

What the Women's Clubs Can Do

Federation of Women's Clubs, often asked her husband, Dr. H. H. Hume, to speak on health matters before her women's club. According to her report on a public health campaign of her home club, "The Beckley Women's Club presented to the people of that section an excellent health program [at which] the laity received health knowledge which proves of marked benefit." The key speaker was the health officer of the county, her husband.[45] Gazelle Hume was granted a position as an expert on health care by the women's voluntary movement in many ways. In 1920, she presented a paper at the Beckley Women's Club entitled "Sketches of Recent Contributions to Medical Surgery."[46] The transference of authority and status from husband to wife was so absolute that she was recognized as an expert in surgery as well as general practice.

Female volunteers were sometimes connected to the medical community through public as well as private ties. The first president of the West Virginia State Nurses' Association, Harriet Camp Lounsberry, was also the first woman to pass the state nurses' registration examination. Her husband, Dr. George Lounsberry, was secretary of the state agency that accepted her credentials.[47] Both of them served on the board of directors of the state Anti-Tuberculosis League.[48] Harriet Camp Lounsberry was a member of the Charleston Women's Club, an affiliate of the West Virginia Federation of Women's Clubs. As president of the state nurses' association, she also served as liaison between that organization and the state federation, with whom the nursing agency associated in 1907.[49]

By spreading the information they acquired in their homes to the community through their voluntary associations, doctors' wives could serve the population at the same time that they supported the presumptions that braced their own social and economic positions. The enthusiasm of women who were not related to medical practitioners was based on a different phenomenon. As medical consumers themselves, middle-class women were convinced of the virtues of scientific treatment and of their obligation to share these advantages with less affluent women in their communities.

Female reformers expressed a growing conviction that physicians could offer important advantages they fervently desired. Clubwomen recognized that through scientific medicine they and their families could experience longer and more secure lives. The validation of the germ theory of disease and the increasing reliance on vaccinations to prevent communicable illness further demonstrated to middle-class women the benefits dispensed through scientific care.[50] Along with this belief in the direct consequences improved medical care could have for their families, clubwomen also imbibed a rhetoric of middle-class domesticity predicated in part on the scientific perspective of the day. To be a good mother, Molly Ladd-Taylor has argued, a woman had to embrace both scientific medicine and scientific mothering.[51]

Some clubwomen developed a reliance on science through their personal education. For the few clubwomen like Jean Dillon and Harriet Camp Lounsberry who trained as nurses, or the even fewer clubwomen like Harriet Jones of West Virginia educated as doctors, scientific medicine was a tangible product with which they were intimately familiar.[52] Although most clubwomen were not formally educated in medicine, some did possess postsecondary training that introduced them to the intellectual structures that guided and defined science. They might have lacked any real knowledge of science, but they knew of its importance and its rising authority.

Bethea Brouse Black, the first woman from southern West Virginia to serve as president of the West Virginia Federation of Women's Clubs, completed two years of college in Pennsylvania before she married and moved to Bluefield in 1894.[53] Mary Belle Lorentz Starcher of Ohio graduated from West Liberty State Normal School, attended West Virginia University, then moved with her husband to Logan County, West Virginia, where he pursued a career as a company doctor. After enrolling at Southern Methodist University in her hometown of Dallas, Texas, for a time, Helen Davis Holcombe followed her husband into the coalfields of Logan County, West Virginia. A native of Iowa, Norma Snodgrass Hogshead met her husband while both of them were students at Valparaiso University in Indiana; they moved to southern West Virginia after World War I.[54]

Besides these women from outside the region, local clubwomen also received college training. Minnie Laura Harris Rutherford was born in eastern Kentucky in 1880 and attended Morris Harvey College in Barboursville, West Virginia, and Millersburg College in Millersburg, Kentucky. She met her future husband, A. G. Rutherford, while they were both attending a "teachers' normal summer school" at White Post, Kentucky, in 1896.[55] Effie Godfrey, whose family was part of the preindustrial elite near Matoaka, West Virginia, graduated from Sullins College in Bristol, Virginia, before she married J. H. Bird in 1907.[56]

Clubwomen's belief in the advances of medical science was

strengthened by the technology doctors were introducing to relieve the discomforts of childbirth. Through increased reliance on sedatives, more frequent use of surgical intervention to shorten labor, and the promotion of the expectation that delivery would occur in the hospital instead of in the home, physicians fundamentally altered the childbirth process during the late nineteenth and early twentieth centuries.[57] These medical strategies were based on the assumption that childbirth was a dangerous event that required medical intervention, reducing pregnant women to patients and encouraging their dependence on physicians.[58]

Appalachian clubwomen imbibed the same lessons their more urban sisters learned. By the 1910s, physicians were opening hospitals in mountain towns to provide childbirth facilities for middle-class women.[59] During the 1920s, doctors in growing communities like Bluefield and Princeton, West Virginia, began to identify themselves as specialists in obstetrics in an attempt to win the allegiance of women who sought treatment by physicians specially trained in childbirth and delivery.[60] Hospitals also promoted this trend by shaping their policies to suit parturient patients.[61] Finally, articles by regional writers in magazines like *Mountain Life and Work* described hospitals as the only appropriate setting for childbirth, reassuring women that "even the banker's wife" would not get better care in the hospital than the care they would receive.[62]

Throughout the nation, women embraced their role as patients of the scientific medical profession, enthusiastically deferring to physicians as the final arbiters of appropriate preventive and curative treatments. Their acceptance of this position also influenced the objectives of their social reform policies. Women were convinced that subordination to a scientifically educated physician was the only way to protect the health of their families and communities. To share the benefits of improved medical care and better health with other women, clubwomen concluded that it was their duty to convince them to acquiesce to the educated medical profession. Clubwomen insisted that, by ceding personal responsibility for one's own health to the judgment of an educated physician, all women, and their families by extension, would prosper.[63]

World War I brought women's concerns about the nation's health to the attention of the broader public. During the conflict, the U.S. military rejected many draftees because they suffered from disabilities caused by childhood illnesses that could have been easily prevented by medical care. Having agitated for public interest in health topics, women activists took advantage of the medical crisis revealed by the war to bolster their position as authorities on the subject. When the war was over, the GFWC's Division of Health renewed its public health campaign. Through its Department of Public Welfare, the national federation directed and supported local clubs that pursued health care projects.[64]

The war increased women's anxiety about the health of American citizens, but it also shaped the tactics they used to respond to the crisis. Women employed militaristic language to warn each other that "the nation's womanhood must defend the nation's health" and that "if American stability is to survive, then the health of our people must be our first consideration."[65] A promotional poster made available to Appalachian clubs depicts a knight on a white horse fighting a dragon who is spewing "disease," "vermin," and "sloth," implying that the public's health could be improved by the defeat of these moral enemies, a campaign that could be led by clubwomen but would only be successful if embraced by the poor and uneducated.[66]

Disease became a tangible enemy not just of the individual but also of the community and the nation. Wellness, therefore, became a prerequisite for democracy in the eyes of American clubwomen, for only through the preservation of a healthy polity could the nation persevere.[67] To protect the family's health and prepare children to be active, intelligent members of society, clubwomen proclaimed "every home a health center."[68] Women were expected to encourage in their own families and in those of their neighbors an awareness of the need "to create a new constructive conception of health."[69]

The members of the GFWC, like physicians, insisted that the public's well-being could be protected only through the "dissemination of accurate scientific knowledge."[70] Although such a mandate gave local clubwomen a general paradigm to emulate, they lacked specific instructions to guide them in their daily work. For assistance in determining the appropriate behavior and actions, female volunteers looked to local physicians.

In an article in the *Quarterly Bulletin of the West Virginia Department of Health*, Mrs. George P. Boomsliter raised the issue of women's organizations' interest in public health. Boomsliter admonished that "the local groups of all the women's organizations are willing to do their share, but they do not know just what needs to be done or how to do it."[71] To find out "what needs to be done" and to legitimize their decisions, clubwomen constantly sought the advice of educated physicians.

Aware of the value of scientific medicine but unable to apply it themselves, clubwomen depended on the expertise of educated physicians. The chairperson of the Division of Public Health of the West Virginia Federation of Women's Clubs chided her colleagues for occasionally failing to "receive trained guidance" because she argued that it undermined the health work of the organization.[72] According to a Virginia clubwoman, medicine represented "new magic" and female volunteers were responsible for bringing the message of these discoveries to the community as directed by the educated physician.[73] When members of the Virginia Federation of Women's Clubs met to discuss a project aimed at aiding disabled children, they reassured their fellow club members that the state board of health and the state medical association had previously approved their work.[74]

Female volunteers promised to defer to and obey physicians, yet some doctors expressed reservations about the wisdom of involving women in campaigns to improve health conditions. Published letters from male practitioners to their colleagues trivialized women's work and encouraged doctors to assign female volunteers only simple tasks, urging local public health officials to give "these ladies plenty to do, for they love to see their names in print."[75] Other physicians exhibited an explicitly misogynistic attitude toward women, questioning their commitment to health reform and denying their claim to any authority on the topic, an attitude that ultimately influenced relations between clubwomen and doctors.[76]

The enthusiasm of the majority of practitioners superseded the reservations of these few opponents, however, and doctors were increasingly willing to form alliances with women volunteers. As early as 1910, physicians in West Virginia recognized the important role that members of women's clubs could play in promulgating the message of scientific medicine to the public. In his presidential address to the West Virginia State Medical Association that year, Dr. T. W. Moore asked his colleagues why so little attention had been directed toward cultivating a close relationship with the women's clubs of the state. He reminded them of the important work done by members of the Kentucky Federation of Women's Clubs after they joined with their state board of health and state medical association to promote public health initiatives in the Bluegrass state.[77]

In Kentucky, Dr. J. A. Stucky, a Lexington physician who volunteered at clinics in the mountain region of the state, expressed his approval of the medical profession's decision "to take the public into its confidence. Its purpose is to make the people a partner in the conservation of health." Women volunteers, he asserted, were pivotal to this ambition since "the woman is just coming into her own" and could serve as the bridge connecting scientific medicine to the general population.[78]

The West Virginia Board of Health agreed with Stucky, offering an appeal entitled "What the Women's Clubs Can Do" in a 1915 publication. The *Quarterly Bulletin of the West Virginia State Board of Health* informed its readers that "the Women's Clubs in the United States are now an enormous power, and they are growing more powerful in the civic and social betterment of this country. If we can disseminate among the women of our land the facts regarding obstetrics, they will raise an undeniable clamor for good obstetricians." The article concluded with the proclamation that alliances between clubwomen and physicians could eliminate midwives and other alternative healers by elevating the standard of care demanded by all women, both rural and urban.[79]

In agreement about the strategy as well as the goals of their campaign, physicians and clubwomen allied to sponsor clinics and public speeches at which physicians argued for the increased reliance of all citizens on educated physicians.[80] In Kentucky, the state board of health devoted one issue of its bulletin a year to the women's clubs. In its 1913 offering, an article entitled "Co-operation of State Board of Health and Kentucky Women's Clubs" described the relationship between women volunteers and physicians and acknowledged the importance of female boosters in promoting modern standards and applications of medicine across the state.[81]

Clubwomen initiated a plethora of innovative projects aimed at improving public health by promoting greater reliance of laypeople on scientific medicine. One of their most popular programs was National Baby Week, which originated in 1916. By encouraging women to bring their babies to clinics where their health would be evaluated, clubwomen and physicians created an opportunity to teach them about proper child care and arouse their enthusiasm for scientific medicine.[82]

Appalachian clubwomen were particularly convinced of the usefulness of baby competitions in coal-mining camps. Since in these camps many working-class families lived in close proximity to one another, clubwomen hoped to play on their competitive natures as well as to encourage them to assist one another in preparing for the contest. The prizes offered in such competitions were often insignificant, but working-class women took part in order to improve their children's health and compete for the honor of being deemed successful mothers by the scientific medical community and middle-class clubwomen.[83]

Clubwomen frequently demonstrated the patronizing attitudes they sometimes exhibited in the better-baby campaigns in other projects they initiated to aid miners and their families. Like volunteers who offered aid to rural blacks in the Deep South, Appalachian clubwomen saw their clients as deficient and potentially harmful to themselves and their children.[84] Without assistance from outside forces, clubwomen reasoned, the miners would continue to live in squalid, unsanitary conditions.[85]

The Women's Club of Omar, West Virginia, offers a unique example of the ways in which middle-class women's suspicions about working-class people's behavior could shape their reform efforts. A mining town in Logan County, Omar was controlled by the West Virginia Coal and Coke Company, which owned the mines that employed the community's workers. In 1926, the wives of the mine operators and other middle-class residents of the town joined together to form the Women's Club of Omar. Since these women were so intimately tied to the men who commanded the town, they were "authorized as its Welfare and Civic Improvement Department." This arrangement so impressed the state federation that it devoted significant attention to it in its *Annual Report*.[86]

With the company's support, the Women's Club of Omar quickly set about establishing agencies and programs to train the camp's women to be good mothers who relied on the scientific advice of experts. Within six months of its creation, the club had acquired its own headquarters, a facility that housed two nurseries, a clinic overseen by the company doctors and staffed by nurses, and a library. To facilitate its health program, the club secured the services of "four graduate nurses, one public health nurse, and one trained social worker."[87]

The nursing staff was kept busy meeting the needs of the miners and their families. Over the winter of 1926–27, the nurses visited and prepared case histories on more than 2,500 families who lived in the mining camps around Omar. In December alone, they made more than 128 home visits to the sick.[88] Five years later, the Omar Women's Club retained responsibility for the health of mining-camp residents. The clubwomen insisted that they had to do so because the miners and their wives continued to embrace unhealthy and "degenerate lifestyles."[89]

Clubwomen sought to improve their local communities and uplift working-class women, but mountain settlement workers generally initiated their projects in rural districts far from their original homes. Clubwomen, as the examination of the Bluefield Women's Club demonstrated and scrutiny of the membership list of any club affirms, were typically middle class and married.[90] Settlement workers, however, were frequently members of wealthy families and single. Many settlement workers were formally educated and had reaped the benefits of college training and extensive travel.[91] They shared clubwomen's belief that females were responsible for the welfare of children and women, but their attitudes were shaped by their class origins and their social and economic positions.

The women who founded the mountain settlement schools were vigorous female reformers who rejected the restrictions of women's traditional domestic sphere and instead sought to assume a greater role in American political life by employing those domestic skills in the construction of new professions.[92] Suffrage was an obvious goal for these women, but they also invested significant energy in efforts to improve conditions for the poor and the socially and physically vulnerable.[93] Like clubwomen, they demanded that the government play a more active role in protecting the home by promoting programs aimed at assisting women and children, a demand that demonstrated their endorsement of the "domestication of politics."[94]

Mountain settlement workers shared the social concerns of clubwomen, but they also actively pursued personal satisfaction from their benevolence work. Single women activists, unlike married clubwomen, were not bound to homes and families but enjoyed what Mary Breckinridge has termed a "wide neighborhood."[95] For example, Linda Neville, an activist who championed antiblindness work in the mountains and made a professional career for herself in the process, ran her own school and was employed by the Lexington Board of Associated Charities before she devoted herself entirely to the antiblindness campaign.[96] Mary Breckinridge, founder of the Frontier Nursing Service, worked for the Children's Bureau during World War I and later traveled to France to serve as a volunteer with the American Committee for Devastated France.[97]

These accomplished women saw the need to improve conditions in the mountains as both a responsibility and an opportunity. As

What the Women's Clubs Can Do

well-educated, often independent women, settlement workers pursued their own reform ambitions separate from the concerns of husbands or dependents. As Robyn Muncy has documented, settlement workers and other women who sought professional legitimacy for their reform efforts campaigned to improve their clients' lives at the same time that they struggled to elevate the status of the institutions and professions they established to ameliorate those conditions.[98]

Clubwomen used their voluntary associations as vehicles to help solidify their claims to middle-class standing. By aiding locals who needed medical attention or other forms of relief, female volunteers could cast themselves as Ladies Bountiful helping the masses. Settlement workers, whose identities were defined in larger contexts, however, were motivated by their perception of Appalachian otherness. Disconnected from the industrial processes that enriched the families of clubwomen and lacking an identification as residents of the region, settlement workers characterized mountain residents as "noble remnants of an Anglo-Saxon, pioneer American culture" who were worthy of relief.[99]

As Jane Becker has demonstrated, the curricula of the mountain settlement schools were defined by the founders' belief that Appalachian people were "backward primitives."[100] To ameliorate the degraded conditions they perceived when visiting rural communities, women reformers modeled their institutions on the urban settlement movement of the late nineteenth century. The urban movement was initiated in London and was heralded by the founding of Toynbee Hall in 1884 by a group of Oxford University students. These programs, which aimed at uplifting the impoverished through social outreach, hinged on the close interaction between the educated elite and the working-class poor. Through this intimacy, created by the establishment of settlement schools in poor neighborhoods, the lower classes would be enlightened and gradually elevated to a more prosperous position in society.[101]

American idealists were attracted to the settlement house model and quickly imported it to the United States. Although initiated in New York City in 1887, its most famous proponent was Jane Addams, founder of Chicago's Hull House.[102] Addams, whose great success with the Hull House popularized the settlement movement, was associated with an astonishing group of women activists who came to be identified with a number of progressive reform movements. Addams and her associates created a uniquely feminine reform community, a model that was emulated in settlements across the United States.[103]

As the urban settlement movement was blossoming, women outside the major metropolitan areas began to discuss the possibility of applying the principle to rural communities. Also influenced by the industrial school model of the post–Civil War era, reformers combined the two paradigms to create institutions that offered both practical training and the moral and educational uplift inherent in the settlement school ideal.[104]

Such an agenda was, by definition, shaped by the values of those who ran the institutions, and scholars have asserted that reformers sought to impart their own class presumptions to rural mountaineers. Karen Tice, however, has convincingly argued that settlement workers were forced by circumstances and inclination to negotiate their agendas with mountain residents. Whether engaged in overt social control or in an evolving discourse with those they sought to aid, settlement workers attempted to prepare their clients to receive the coming industrial order by teaching them work skills and promoting an attachment to scientific principles. They pursued a campaign to educate those who were "perceived to be defective mothers [and] targeted as needing the instruction of reformers to ensure good nutritional, health and child-rearing practices."[105]

The settlement schools established at Hindman and Pine Mountain in eastern Kentucky offered the most significant application of these principles and ambitions in Appalachia and became the standards for rural settlement programs in the mountains. In addition to striving to educate and uplift eastern Kentucky's people, settlement workers became the key conveyors of the principles of modern, scientific medicine into the highlands of Appalachia.

The settlement movement in eastern Kentucky was intimately associated with the careers of Katherine Pettit and May Stone. Pettit, a native of the Lexington area, was descended from "pioneer stock, both sides," according to her 1936 obituary in the Pine Mountain Settlement School newsletter.[106] Stone, who was born in Owingsville, Kentucky, moved with her family to Louisville as an adolescent before attending Wellesley College.[107]

Pettit and Stone exemplified the rising number of single, educated females who, in the post–Civil War era, sought meaningful work in the public sphere. Active members of their churches, they both supported home missionary work and other benevolent causes. They also committed themselves to various women's voluntary associa-

What the Women's Clubs Can Do

tions, wearing the label "clubwoman" before taking on the mantle of "settlement worker."

As David Whisnant has observed in his study of the Kentucky settlement movement, Katherine Pettit was a private woman and little is known about her early life after she completed her education at the Sayre Female Institute in Lexington in 1887. One thing that is certain is that she was actively involved in the Women's Christian Temperance Union and other female voluntary associations, affiliations that provided her with formal allies and give us with some idea of her activities and beliefs before she initiated her work in eastern Kentucky.[108] Both Pettit and Stone were affiliated with the Kentucky Federation of Women's Clubs, and it was at the association's 1899 convention that the women initiated steps that culminated in the creation of the Hindman Settlement School.[109]

During the last few years of the nineteenth century, a number of outsiders, including missionaries, ballad collectors, and writers, traveled throughout the mountains of eastern Kentucky seeking to uplift, preserve, or romanticize the mountaineers. Pettit joined this ensemble in 1895 when she visited the isolated communities of Perry County, a journey that she recalled took three days from Lexington, one by train and two by wagon. For the next several years, she returned each summer to offer assistance to the residents of Hazard and other mountain communities by bringing the "traveling libraries of the State W.C.T.U. and the State Federation of Women's Clubs."[110]

By 1899, the Kentucky Federation of Women's Clubs was convinced that aid beyond the mere distribution of library books was necessary to elevate eastern Kentucky's citizens. At the association's assembly that year, Pettit proposed the establishment of a settlement school to educate and uplift the natives. The clubwomen received her suggestion enthusiastically, and Stone, the state federation secretary, volunteered to help administer the project.[111]

Pettit, Stone, and their associates offered programs at a camp outside Hazard in the summer of 1899. A group of citizens who lived on Troublesome Creek convinced the women to move their project to Hindman, a smaller village, the next summer. Encouraged by the enthusiasm of Hindman's residents, who offered land, materials, and labor for the construction of a permanent settlement house and school, Pettit and Stone agreed to establish a settlement outside the village. The resources and support offered by the locals were critical to the project's inception and success, but Pettit and

Stone realized that their venture required an infusion of hard currency, a commodity that many mountain residents lacked.[112]

Pettit and Stone initiated a fund-raising campaign to collect the necessary cash to inaugurate the programs they envisioned offering at the Hindman Settlement School. To secure the required capital, they turned to their old allies in the women's club movement. By addressing chapters of various female organizations such as the Women's Christian Temperance Union, Pettit and Stone gained the financial support they needed to open the Hindman Settlement School in the summer of 1902. Lucy Furman, a contemporary of Pettit and Stone, wrote that although they realized their tactics were "incredible to modern publicity-hounds," they insisted that limiting their initial campaign to audiences composed primarily of women's clubs was the only way to avoid exploiting the highlanders. They were convinced by their lengthy association with women's groups that they could rely on their colleagues not to capitalize on the mountaineers' plight.[113]

The staff at Hindman and their colleagues at the Pine Mountain Settlement School, a separate institution established by Pettit in Letcher County in 1911, considered the introduction of scientific medical care and scientific knowledge a key component of their mission to improve the lives of mountain people.[114] The Hindman Settlement School employed its first nurse in 1904, just two years after the facility opened. Pine Mountain always maintained a nursing staff as well. By the middle of the 1920s, both settlements had in-patient clinics and the school at Hindman was outfitted with an operating room. As a reflection of their desire to improve the general conditions of life in the mountains, the settlements also offered out-patient clinics for nonstudents.[115]

Workers at Hindman and Pine Mountain, as well as those at other settlements that sprang up in the mountains after the turn of the century, often looked to their allies in the women's clubs for aid when arranging for special clinics held by independent physicians from outside the region. The most notable example of the cooperation that developed between settlement workers, clubwomen, and physicians can be found in the work of Dr. J. A. Stucky, an otolaryngologist who led the campaign to eradicate trachoma in eastern Kentucky.

Recognized as a successful specialist in Lexington, Stucky began his work in eastern Kentucky in 1910 when he accepted the invitation of H. S. Murdock, a minister who directed a mission in Buck-horn, in Perry County, Kentucky, to investigate the prevalence of trachoma among the mountain people. By 1911, however, Stucky had shifted his work to the Hindman Settlement School, and in 1922, he moved his clinics to the more remote settlement at Pine Mountain.[116]

Stucky held clinics for general medical care and the treatment of trachoma at the settlement schools on an annual or biannual basis. At these clinics, Stucky and his assistants examined countless patients and performed extremely high numbers of operations, often moving patients who were recovering from anesthesia outside in order to prepare for the next surgery.[117] Because of the massive publicity given to the trachoma epidemic, the federal government eventually intervened and established state-supported trachoma hospitals in Hindman, Hyden, Jackson, London, Pikeville, and Greenville. By 1928, all but one of these treatment centers had closed, and trachoma had become an uncommon ailment in eastern Kentucky.[118]

Stucky depended on settlement workers to facilitate his campaigns to improve the health of mountain residents, but he also relied on aid from clubwomen in the Bluegrass and western portions of Kentucky. Like Stone and Pettit, Stucky received significant fiscal, social, and civic support from Kentucky's clubwomen. One of his most important allies in the campaign to alleviate trachoma was Linda Neville, a Lexington clubwoman who devoted her career to the fight against preventable blindness in Kentucky.

Linda Neville was born into an affluent family in central Kentucky. After graduating from Bryn Mawr College, she "returned home to devote herself to what was then called 'charity work.'" Neville, whose father had endured an episode of blindness, became absorbed in the fight to prevent the disorder after she met a young mountain woman who had been brought to Lexington to receive treatment to prevent loss of her sight. Sponsored by a clubwoman from the Bluegrass region, the mountain woman inspired Neville to pursue a program to fight blindness in eastern Kentucky.[119]

In order to discover more about conditions in the mountains, Neville contacted Pettit and Stone at the Hindman Settlement School. As upper-class natives of the Bluegrass region and fellow Kentucky Federation of Women's Clubs members, Stone and Pettit had much in common with Neville, who was personally acquainted

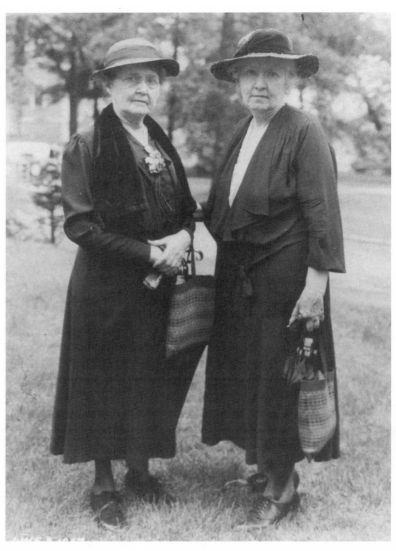

Settlement supporters like Lucy Furman (left) and Linda Neville (right) also shared ties to various women's clubs. Audio-Visual Archives, Special Collections and Archives, University of Kentucky Libraries.

with them and their work. In 1908, Neville went to Hindman to inspect the school's health programs to gather ideas for the campaign to avert preventable blindness.[120]

When she returned from the mountains, Neville followed the path blazed by Pettit and Stone, and later emulated by Mary Breckinridge, by turning to members of local women's organizations for

What the Women's Clubs Can Do

support. Their donations provided the basis for the Mountain Fund for Needy Eye Sufferers.[121] Although this project was initially quite small, it served as the genesis of the more substantial Kentucky Society for the Prevention of Blindness.[122]

The Kentucky Federation of Women's Clubs played a pivotal role in promoting the creation of the Kentucky Society for the Prevention of Blindness. Neville, whose work through the Mountain Fund had gained recognition outside Kentucky, was approached by Dr. F. Park Lewis of the American Medical Association and Louisa Schuyler, head of the Russell Sage Foundation's Committee on the Prevention of Blindness, about establishing a state association to promote the prevention of blindness. With their support, and with the blessing of Dr. J. N. McCormack, the chair of the Kentucky Board of Health, Neville proceeded with her project.[123]

To bring these plans to fruition, Neville returned to her old allies in the volunteer movement. At the 1910 convention of the Kentucky Federation of Women's Clubs in Frankfort, Neville sought support for an antiblindness association. The clubwomen responded enthusiastically, and Neville quickly gathered the names of twenty-five prominent members who offered their assistance in her campaign. These women, primarily citizens of Louisville, demonstrated the federation's continued strength in the western and central areas of the state as well as its persistent interest in the problems of Appalachian Kentucky.[124]

Having won support from the state federation, Neville used her ties with the association to create opportunities for fund-raising at the local level. She pressured her colleagues in various women's associations by seeking invitations "to clubs, missionary societies, meetings, and banquets and . . . insisting on telling what is going on in unknown parts of Kentucky."[125]

Neville also made use of the Kentucky Federation of Women's Clubs' alliance with the state board of health. As a chairperson of a standing committee of the state federation, Neville convinced other clubwomen of the importance of the antiblindness campaign. The federation acknowledged the significance of Neville's work by featuring it in articles it sponsored in the *Bulletin of the State Board of Health of Kentucky*. The April 1913 issue urged clubwomen to push for legislation to mandate the use of proper "scientific methods" by obstetricians to prevent blindness. A headline in that issue advised, "Kentucky Clubs! Help the Mountain Fund!"[126]

Like Neville and her colleagues at the settlement schools, Mary

Breckinridge, the founder of the Frontier Nursing Service, also took advantage of her connections with the women's clubs of Kentucky. Other members of Breckinridge's prestigious, wealthy Kentucky family were affiliated with the club movement and supported the settlement schools. Her kinswomen Sophonisba Breckinridge, Madeline McDowell Breckinridge, and Curry Desha Breckinridge all backed the early settlement movement. Sophonisba Breckinridge, who attended Wellesley with May Stone, provided the Kentucky settlement workers with a direct connection to Jane Addams since she had lived at the Hull House when she was a graduate student at the University of Chicago.[127]

The Breckinridge women, like Stone, Pettit, and Neville, relied on their women's club affiliations to support their work. Madeline McDowell Breckinridge, for example, committed herself to the crusade for educational reform and depended on her colleagues in the Kentucky Federation of Women's Clubs to campaign for progressive improvements in the state's school system.[128]

Mary Breckinridge was driven by maternalist ambitions rooted in personal as well as ideological concerns. After the death of her first husband, the failure of her second marriage, and the deaths of two children, Breckinridge turned her energies away from her own home and toward the larger community. By replacing lay midwives with educated nurse-midwives, Breckinridge believed that she could improve the conditions under which women gave birth and lower the risks of infant and maternal death during childbirth.[129]

Breckinridge was educated as a nurse-midwife in Europe and returned to Kentucky to establish a nurse-midwifery project in the state's eastern mountains. To accomplish this objective, she solicited the backing of important members of the Kentucky Federation of Women's Clubs.[130] The second meeting of the Kentucky Committee for Mothers and Babies, the original name of the Frontier Nursing Service, was held at the home of Mrs. S. C. Henning, in Louisville's elite Cherokee Park neighborhood. A supporter of the women's club movement, Henning was not the only affiliate who assisted Breckinridge in launching her project. In addition to Pettit, Stone, Neville, and a number of her female relatives who were active in the women's club movement, Breckinridge convinced at least three other active clubwomen to serve on the Kentucky Committee for Mothers and Babies.[131]

Clubwomen also provided Breckinridge with critical financial assistance. Through her family and social connections, Breckinridge was introduced to a number of voluntary associations that offered her opportunities for fund-raising and promotional activities. Her ability to gain access to groups like the Kentucky Women's Club of New York enabled her to tap into the extensive resources of women's organizations across the country. These alliances, combined with the ties Breckinridge maintained with benevolent agencies in her home state, furnished her with the necessary funds to supplement her own resources and keep the Frontier Nursing Service afloat financially.[132]

As Theda Skocpol has argued for the nation at large, the Appalachian settlement elite and the middle-class clubwomen who supported them while conducting benevolence projects in their own communities were intimately bound to each other by both practical and ideological ties. Guided by the maternalism that, according to Molly Ladd-Taylor, was the overwhelming ideology among women reformers in this era, clubwomen and settlement workers identified Appalachian mothers and their children as special populations that required salvation through the introduction of modern standards of medical care and disease prevention.[133]

Settlement workers and clubwomen, however, had different views of the people they were determined to save and why they needed to be saved. Clubwomen saw the increasingly impoverished immigrants and African Americans who labored in the coalfields and lived in the coal camps as culpable for their own poverty. Living amid intemperance and filth, coal camp mothers were perceived as in need of uplift and reform. Miners and their families could, in principle, receive medical care from the physicians who worked for the coal companies, but clubwomen still targeted them as a population that needed to be encouraged to embrace and obey the dictates of scientific medicine. Although they did not question the economic paradigms that kept workers in destitution and filth, they did campaign to ameliorate the conditions they believed the workers could change themselves.

The Frontier Nursing Service, Neville's Mountain Fund, and the Hindman and Pine Mountain Settlement Schools, however, all enjoyed great success because they, as Whisnant has documented and Becker has confirmed, offered outsiders the vision of a traditional Anglo-Saxon culture free of modern interference.[134] Although such views ignored the realities of the changes that had already remade Appalachian life, they did legitimize claims such as that of Linda

Neville that mountain mothers were especially worthy of medical assistance because they were the product of a singularly pure Anglo-Saxon heritage.[135]

Although eastern Kentucky mining camps were filling up with immigrants from Europe and African American refugees from the Lower South who challenged their presumptions, settlement activists still held up native Appalachian mountaineers as paragons of breeding handicapped only by their environment and isolation.[136] In his appeals for support of the Mountain Fund, J. A. Stucky informed his readers that "the natives of the Highlands of Kentucky are not in a class with the immigrants, which are the sweepings of Europe, neither are they of the 'slum element,' so well known in our large cities."[137] According to Whisnant, workers at the Hindman Settlement School faced some of their greatest challenges as the mining industry invaded eastern Kentucky and fundamentally altered the traditional landscape, in part through the arrival of outsiders who did not share the Anglo-Saxon heritage so lauded by mountain reformers.[138]

Settlement workers viewed the introduction of scientific medical care as a component of their campaign to assist the mountaineers and couched their efforts in the rhetoric of maternalism and a desire to protect the Anglo-Saxon culture of the mountains. These workers, however, had the power to select which attributes of Appalachian culture were worthy of preservation. Traditional forms of healing and care were not included on their list of desirable features, and workers believed that as soon as mountain mothers discovered that scientific medicine could lower infant and maternal mortality, they would enthusiastically embrace contemporary methods of treating illness and abandon time-honored practices.[139]

The settlement workers, nurses, and doctors who brought modern health care to the mountains were often correct in their expectations, and many of the Kentucky highlanders were delighted by the advantages scientific medicine offered. The settlement schools and medical relief programs filled their promotional literature with anecdotes of the sacrifices mountain people made to acquire medical assistance for members of their families.

But resistance to new medical practices did exist. When settlement workers observed that mothers were reluctant to accept prescribed change, they accused them of having an unhealthy attachment to their children. By dismissing these mothers as "bad mothers," settlement workers could reconcile their own desire to

What the Women's Clubs Can Do

remake mountain life with the obstinacy they sometimes encountered among those they intended to aid.[140]

Convinced of the merits of scientific medicine, clubwomen and settlement workers believed that health care had to be rationalized under the control of educated physicians. The resistance they met from country residents and industrial workers indicated to them that transforming medical care required fundamental changes in patients' expectations and attitudes. To achieve that metamorphosis, clubwomen, settlement workers, and their medical allies initiated a panoply of programs to aid and reeducate mountain dwellers and their more modern cousins in the region's coal camps.

CHAPTER FOUR

Women,

Health Care,

and the

Community

Inspired by their belief that the community was an extension of the home, clubwomen and settlement workers joined physicians in a campaign to promote improved health through a reliance on scientific medicine. In the process of introducing rural mountaineers and industrial workers to the advantages of modern medical care, women's organizations significantly improved the lives and well-being of many mountain residents. By employing public health nurses to educate families about infant and maternal health and to offer public screenings to evaluate women and children for illness, women's organizations became critical transmitters of the new medical system.

As nonprofessionals whose benevolence was based in their domesticity, clubwomen had little real authority to demand reform or support it. To improve community health by promoting scientific medical care, therefore, clubwomen had to negotiate every program with those delivering services as well as those receiving them. Women reformers sought assistance from physicians but could not demand or coerce their cooperation. When dealing with public health nurses, activists were bargaining with another group of workers who were seeking professional status. Unlike doctors, these nurses articulated a feminine model of professionalization that better corresponded with the maternalist goals of women reformers.[1] The similarities of their ideologies, coupled with the economic and social advantages the reformers had over the nurses, eased the relationship but limited the benefits clubwomen offered nurses in their drive to achieve professional status.[2] Finally, no matter what advantages reformers offered to working families, they could not force Appalachian citizens in coal camps and on mountain farms to accept the intellectual presumptions that supported scientific medical care. To win them to those ideals, women reformers had to enter into an exchange with locals, convincing them of the benefits of modern medicine at the same time that they recognized the persistence of older traditions.

Determined to secure whatever legitimacy they could by adhering to the principles of scientific evaluation, both clubwomen and settlement workers initiated their health work by conducting surveys to document local conditions. Such an undertaking linked these Appalachian reformers to colleagues across the country who also investigated their communities in search of potential dangers. Maureen Flanagan has written that women were committed to guarding their neighborhoods in the same way that they were devoted to protecting their homes; by documenting conditions, they sought to acquire the knowledge necessary to defend the welfare of the larger family in which they lived.[3] Settlement workers, who were typically well educated, modeled their surveys on those conducted by agencies such as the Children's Bureau. By striving to make objective evaluations based on quantitative data, they demonstrated that, like Children's Bureau head Julia Lathrop, they believed in the "importance of social research as a sound means of social reform."[4]

Through their surveys, clubwomen and settlement workers discovered that different but related problems plagued the populations they served. Sanitation, nutrition, and hygiene issues were of most immediate concern among coal miners and other industrial workers. In more isolated communities, settlement workers struggled to introduce rural mountaineers to the advantages of regular contact with educated medical providers. They, too, campaigned to inform their clients about sanitation and hygiene, targeting mothers and children as the primary recipients of education and preventive care.

Women reformers needed the assistance of physicians to accomplish this goal, and doctors needed female advocates to promote public acceptance of their professional authority.[5] Physicians, however, were unwilling to allow women reformers to set an independent health reform agenda. When efforts to promote full-time public health units were stalled by doctors' recalcitrance, female reformers came to depend on the services of public health nurses as semiautonomous professionals who could educate and administer care but were reliant on their benefactors, as well as physicians, for legitimacy.

Although tensions sometimes divided women reformers from the public health nurses they employed, this alliance provided mountain residents with a great number of educational and preventive programs.[6] Supported by federal funds through the Sheppard-Towner Act and by continued private donations that funded local clinics, visiting nurses, and settlement school programs, female reformers set out to offer immediate remedies for the deprivation they saw around them. At the same time, as historians Seth Koven and Sonya Michel have argued, "in the name of friendship and in the interests of the health of the family and the nation, these reformers claimed the right to instruct and regulate the conduct of the working-class woman."[7]

The most obvious campaign to remake working-class experience in the mountains was the crusade by middle-class and elite reformers, supported by the nurses they employed and overseen by physicians, to regulate and eventually prohibit the practice of lay midwifery in the mountains. Reformers opposed midwifery for a variety of reasons. For clubwomen, midwives were a symbol of the region's retrogression and its tardiness in fulfilling the promises of the modern industrial economy. In the opinion of many nurses, midwives failed to embrace the professional standards to which nurses aspired, and as potential symbols of the rejection of scientific advancement, they had to be supervised and educated.[8] Physicians shared the nurses' perception of midwifery as a sign of the persistence of prescientific beliefs and as a possible threat to parturient women. They also interpreted the continued existence of midwives as a potential challenge to physicians' coveted monopoly as the only autonomous professionals within the medical community. By eliminating lay midwives, physicians, nurses, and clubwomen could all elevate their own status at the same time that they fulfilled their obligations and aspirations to ameliorate the conditions of disadvantaged mountaineers, satisfying the altruistic as well as the egocentric ambitions that marked the campaign to improve medicine in the mountains.[9]

Before moving against midwives, reformers applied the scientific principles of survey research to document the practice of midwifery and the conditions under which such deliveries occurred. By doing so, they asserted their alleged objectivity and fortified their claims to be pursuing a tangible improvement.[10]

The social survey, widely used by reformers during the Progressive Era, was advertised as an objective tool intended to provide an accurate portrait of the conditions in which rural or working-class people lived and labored. As Kathryn Kish Sklar has described, these surveys were rarely truly impartial, however, and were generally influenced by what she has termed the "moral emphasis" of applied social science research in the Progressive Era. Clubwomen and settlement workers, like reformers across the country, strived for objectivity, but the class and social assumptions that guided their work inevitably affected the outcome of their research.[11]

A number of agencies, both public and private, investigated conditions in rural Appalachia and in the region's coal camps during the Progressive Era and into the New Deal years. The Children's Bureau of the U.S. Department of Labor, for example, prepared studies of a mountain county in Kentucky in 1922 and bituminous coal–mining communities in West Virginia in 1923.[12] Mary Breckinridge, to determine the need for a project like the Frontier Nursing Service, rode across the hills of Leslie, Owsley, and Knott Counties in eastern Kentucky during the summer of 1923 and compiled a lengthy report of her encounters with lay midwives and traditional doctors.[13] Two of her assistants authored subsequent reports, one of which was submitted as a dissertation to Columbia University, granting academic legitimacy to their documentation of the lack of skilled medical care available to rural Kentuckians.[14]

Clubwomen also conducted social surveys and used the information they gathered to demonstrate the need for women's involvement in improving the health of American citizens. From the General Federation of Women's Clubs (GFWC) national clearinghouse, state and local clubs received requests for information about the composition of county or city health units. These comprehensive questionnaires asked for specific information on the number and type of professionals employed and the salaries paid to each. The majority of these surveys sought detailed data on the health of the community, focusing particularly on the epidemiology of specific diseases and the programs initiated to prevent them.[15]

Appalachian clubwomen joined their colleagues across the United States in energetically inspecting the needs of their towns and cities.[16] They were encouraged in this process by their state federations, agencies that copied the GFWC by sending forms to the local clubs soliciting information about the status of health in their communities. In Virginia, this questionnaire included queries on the clubs' health activities as well as community conditions, demonstrating the state federation's expectation that locals would not only chronicle health conditions but also act to improve them.[17] As fortunate women who enjoyed the security of middle-class comfort, Appalachian clubwomen could not be disinterested observers, but "as Anglo-Saxon women of means they had a special aptitude and responsibility to care for the nation's less fortunate children."[18]

Like local reformers, agents of the federal Children's Bureau relied on social science techniques to record the conditions under which children lived in Appalachia. Nettie McGill, the bureau official who authored *The Welfare of Children in the Bituminous Coal Mining Communities in West Virginia* in 1923, described a landscape of isolated mining settlements whose residents faced chronic ill health due to the environmental and social forces that shaped their existence. Mining families lived in inadequate and crowded housing in congested camps. Their homes were seldom equipped with modern sanitation facilities, and garbage and sewage removal was rarely attended to by the companies that owned the miners' houses. Residents also told McGill that they received inconsistent and insufficient health care from the coal company doctors.[19]

The consequences of these circumstances, as a 1917 Metropolitan Life Insurance Company survey confirmed, were not surprising: Appalachian miners and their families suffered exceptionally high rates of typhoid, scarlet fever, tuberculosis, and diphtheria.[20] McGill asserted that unhealthy environmental conditions were allowed to continue because "whether from a lack of time or from a lack of realization of its value to the community, no company doctor had attempted any educational propaganda looking to the prevention of disease and the preservation of health."[21]

Representatives of the U.S. Coal Commission discovered similar conditions when they came to Appalachia in the early 1920s. The commission reported that only nine of the forty-five West Virginia company towns examined achieved a rating of more than 75 percent for adequate medical care. Only eight camps earned a mark of over 75 percent for sanitary sewage disposal, and only six received this rating for decent housing conditions. Statistics reflecting conditions in the coal-producing regions of Kentucky and Virginia, although lumped together with information on the Maryland coalfields, demonstrated that miners and their families there endured conditions similar to those found in West Virginia.[22]

Although conditions were unhealthy, according to the survey,

Women, Health Care, and the Community

residents generally did have access to medical care. Miners who resided in thirty-eight of forty-four independent West Virginia towns with populations under 2,500 could acquire a physician's care. In West Virginia towns with populations between 2,500 and 10,000, all miners could secure aid from local doctors. The same was true in the four towns with more than 10,000 inhabitants.[23]

In rural mountain communities, however, country people were less able to obtain trained medical care. Although those who surveyed nonindustrial rural communities also documented inadequate sanitation, poor housing, and inferior water supplies, they were most alarmed by the continued absence of educated practitioners in rural mountain areas beyond the reach of the new industrial infrastructure. Mary Breckinridge focused on the practice of lay midwifery in her 1923 portrait of eastern Kentucky, but she also commented on the inadequacy of some of the mountain dwellings and the lack of hygiene among their inhabitants.[24] W. Bertram Ireland, an employee of the Frontier Nursing Service, noted that there were only four indoor toilets in Leslie County, Kentucky, in 1926 and that contagious diseases such as typhoid, hookworm, diarrhea, and "sores are pitifully prevalent in summer time. Add to this the fact that there is not a registered physician in the county and no guess can compute the distress and disablement."[25]

Social surveys proved to clubwomen and settlement workers alike that medical care was an issue that had to be addressed if living standards were to be raised among Appalachia's less affluent and more isolated residents. These two groups of reformers, however, faced different concerns as they organized to promote scientific medicine among their selected clienteles. Clubwomen realized that medical services were within the physical reach of those who lived in mining or timbering camps but that workers had to be convinced of the value of trained medical care. Settlement workers faced the more direct need of simply securing skilled care for country people, who seldom enjoyed access to a trained physician.

Appalachian women activists were unable to achieve these goals by themselves.[26] Without formal medical credentials, women reformers had no legitimacy in this arena. Increasingly wed to the ideals of science, women looked to doctors to guide them in their campaign to improve the conditions of women and children in the mountains.[27] Physicians, who stood to further their economic and social ambitions by intensifying and expanding their relationship with the working classes and rural farmers, were only too happy to oblige. In essence, doctors could increase their market by promoting an awareness of scientific medicine among populations that had not yet developed an intimate dependence on its advantages.

In mining communities, new medical ideals were embodied in the company physician. To ensure the stability of their workforce and, according to historian David Corbin, to increase the dependence of the laborers on the operators, companies deducted a fee from their workers' checks that was devoted to paying for a doctor's services for the entire mining community.[28]

This system offered some benefit to the miners and their families, but it did not guarantee extensive or high quality care for all residents.[29] As allies of the company owners and ambitious professionals seeking to secure their own financial and social positions, many physicians provided only minimal care through their company positions.[30] Their actions did little to encourage confidence in educated practitioners and sometimes discouraged reliance on the medical profession. Female advocates of the professional medical model said little publicly about the inequalities of the company doctor system, but their records suggest that they realized that the actions of a few unscrupulous physicians could undermine the advancement of health care among the poorer classes.[31]

Clubwomen, lacking the authority to comment on relations between company doctors and patients, directed their efforts toward advocating for increased public health activity. Through public health screenings and preventive programs, women could work to protect the welfare of mothers and children without challenging the company doctor, who was, in some cases, married to a member of the club. By working under the supervision of and in association with the doctor, clubwomen could improve conditions for workers and maintain their allegiance to the established social order at the same time.

To improve health conditions in coal settlements and growing commercial towns, clubwomen created a plethora of educational and preventive projects. Local iterations of national projects included sanitation campaigns, pre- and postnatal clinics, vaccinations, well-baby and child evaluations, and antituberculosis work.[32] Many of these projects were tremendously successful and promoted the public image of the women's clubs as important agitators for community health. In Bluefield, West Virginia, for example, the local club created so much enthusiasm for its public health campaign that the city eventually assumed responsibility for funding its work on a full-time basis.[33] The Virginia Federation of Women's Clubs proudly proclaimed that, although it was not completely responsible for every public health effort in Appalachian Virginia, "whenever it seemed necessary for our clubs to step in and lend a helping hand they have done so."[34]

Appalachian clubwomen worked to promote public health programs at both the state and the local levels. They campaigned for the passage of laws requiring the registration of births and deaths with state governments; without such legislation, the West Virginia federation asserted, "the state cannot progress in health matters."[35] In Kentucky, organizations such as the Owingsville Women's Club sent telegrams to the state legislature when it threatened to reduce the state board of health's funding and autonomy.[36] The Virginia Federation of Women's Clubs resolved that "public health work should be as fully incorporated into our government as is public education."[37] The Division of Public Welfare of the West Virginia Federation of Women's Clubs made agitation for a full-time county health unit one of its principal goals for 1922.[38] The Prestonsburg, Kentucky, Women's Club was established in 1919 when a number of local women banned together to campaign for the creation of a public health office.[39]

Clubwomen were guided by the presumption that they were working to build full-time local public health offices that would be directed by educated physicians. The premise that educated, typically male physicians would oversee the programs established by the women's clubs was espoused by the GFWC and embraced by its subordinates and was tremendously influential in shaping club efforts in the public health arena.[40]

Across the region, Appalachian clubwomen joined colleagues from the non-Appalachian portions of their states to promote the employment of physicians to oversee public health activities. West Virginia's clubwomen, in their magazine articles and yearly reports, were emphatic that doctors should head health units.[41] In their effort to encourage the employment of physicians in the public health offices of their state, Kentucky clubwomen promoted higher salaries for such agents. The state medical association offered these clubwomen public thanks in the *Kentucky Medical Journal* in an article that praised their efforts toward "creating the proper public sentiment."[42]

Clubwomen did not possess the political clout to convince the state or county government to provide funding for public health units in every county or town.[43] Independent physicians often opposed campaigns to establish public health units. Some county governments, hesitant to raise taxes to fund such projects, also rejected efforts to promote public health agencies.[44] Finally, many physicians contended that public health programs targeted at coal camps were redundant since contract physicians were employed to deliver preventive as well as curative treatments there.[45] When they were unable to secure the employment of physicians to oversee public health work on a full-time basis, Appalachian reformers followed the model being developed across the nation by other women's groups and employed public health nurses.[46] A club associate summed up the attitude toward this prospect when she advised in the *West Virginia Clubwoman*: "If it is not possible to bring about a public opinion which will insist upon [the employment of a physician], try for a public health nurse."[47]

Employment of a trained nurse protected the clubwomen from physicians' criticism that they were acting "without securing [direction] from recognized authorities."[48] At the same time, public health nurses were often employees of the women's clubs and, as such, were prohibited from gaining too much autonomy by their subordination to both their employers and the physicians who cooperated with the clubs to implement the programs.[49]

For public health nurses, who were seeking to secure professional status in their own right, employment by a benevolent association was both a curse and a blessing. As nursing historians Karen Buhler-Wilkerson, Susan Armeny, and Barbara Melosh have demonstrated, the autonomy secured by public health nurses through their employment by women's groups enhanced their independence, but it led them away from the hospital, which physicians were increasingly insisting was the most appropriate place for nurses to practice.[50]

Unlike women volunteers, who saw their work as benevolent, public health workers were struggling to achieve full professional status and to protect their own economic and social interests. Because of their relatively autonomous work environment, public health nurses had the greatest opportunity of practitioners of any nursing specialty to achieve full professional legitimacy before World War II.[51] To pursue that ambition, Appalachian public health nurses accepted employment from middle-class clubwomen and used the clubwomen's social prestige to advance their own efforts to gain professional recognition.

The employment of public health nurses by women's clubs was

common across the United States, and clubwomen were fundamental in promoting the independence of educated nurses.[52] In Appalachia, clubwomen employed nurses to accomplish a myriad of goals. The Beckley, West Virginia, Women's Club hired a nurse to inspect and inoculate children in the Raleigh County schools. Similar work assignments were undertaken by nurses in Radford, Virginia, and other locations across the region.[53] Some nurses held "Health Crusades" for children, "a plan for teaching hygiene which, in turn, teaches health."[54]

In addition to their more conventional duties, nurses were given direct responsibility for the social development of their vulnerable clients. Like public health nurses elsewhere, Appalachian nurses were expected to "bring a message with their medicine."[55] The Bluefield, West Virginia, Women's Club sent twenty underprivileged girls, "under care of a special nurse, for one week to a YWCA camp."[56] Natalie Rudd, a public health nurse for the Bramwell, West Virginia, Women's Club, taught maternal and infant hygiene courses to local women. She was also charged with accompanying them to the first annual meeting of the Maternal and Infant Hygiene Association in Mercer County in 1924.[57] The Radford Women's Club went so far as to command its public health nurse to distribute rose plants to "the colored women in town."[58]

Such missions remind us that public health nurses and their allies were engaged in more than health care when they initiated projects in country communities and mining districts. Nurses, combining a commitment to science with a commitment to a culture of reform based on middle-class standards of parenting and family life, were agents of morality as well as health when they entered working-class homes. Like other new helping professions, nurses, acting for the middle-class women who employed them, attempted to redefine good mothering for working-class mothers.[59] When judging the quality of their clients' home lives, nurses reflected both the "values of women's culture" and a commitment to the principles of science that increasingly defined acceptable parenting.[60]

As recognized agents of scientific medicine, nurses, through programs sponsored by clubwomen, attempted to teach patients who attended clinics in coal and timber villages about their appropriate role in the medical structure. Inhabitants of coal camps and settled communities already had some exposure to the modern, hierarchical medical system, but clubwomen and nurses constantly reminded them of their subordinate status as patients in the new health care paradigm. To impart this lesson, the West Virginia Federation of Women's Clubs sponsored lectures by physicians on "when to call a doctor."[61] The *Virginia Club Woman*, the magazine of the Virginia federation, sold copies of a playlet entitled "The Federation Clinic" that could be used to teach citizens about the workings of the health care system and their role in that structure.[62] To formalize the inequality of these relationships, nurses in rural Virginia were instructed to wear "some striking and becoming uniform" to set them apart and encourage the citizens to respect and obey their directives.[63]

Nurses shouldered extensive and diverse responsibilities, but they were not granted reasonable financial compensation. Clubs that employed public health nurses clearly viewed their relationship with the nurses as one between employer and employee. Nurses were hired on a temporary basis and seldom enjoyed secure employment, sometimes accepting positions with women's clubs that lasted less than six months. At times, nurses were hired on an as-needed basis, being called to work at particular clinics or educational events and then dismissed as soon as the work was complete, combining the economic model of private-duty nursing with the innovative new public health paradigm.[64]

Even nurses who enjoyed the goodwill of their employers and whose services were highly valued were often vulnerable since clubs frequently had few resources with which to pay them. In order to maintain their local public health nurse in 1924, the women's clubs of Bluefield and Princeton, West Virginia, were forced to combine their available capital and solicit matching aid from an outside source. The women's clubs raised their contribution to this fund by holding an annual Christmas Seal campaign and spring Daisy Day sale.[65] The clubwomen of Bluefield and Princeton were not alone in their reliance on the generosity of their fellow citizens. Since clubwomen were seldom employed outside their own homes, they had little disposable cash to contribute toward the public health work they initiated and were forced to hold fund-raising events to support public health nurses.[66]

This concern over payment of public health nurses illustrates a significant difference between doctors and nurses in the eyes of women volunteers. Doctors, whose social and economic status was much higher than that of nurses, were seldom "employed" by clubwomen. Physicians "volunteered" their time or "offered aid" to those unfortunate enough to need public health assistance.[67] Nurses, however, were "employed" or "hired" and were clearly seen as

Women, Health Care, and the Community

employees. They depended on the financial benefits of the job and therefore were seldom able to contribute to the work as charitable volunteers.[68] The language of benevolence used to describe doctors and clubwomen was denied to public health nurses, whose economic and social status placed them outside that tradition.

Nurses were perceived and treated as employees and not charitable agents, but they did obtain a number of benefits from their relationship with the clubwomen who employed them. The first and most obvious advantage was the financial support they gained by finding an appropriate market for their skills. Unlike private-duty or hospital nurses, public health nurses sought employment in a burgeoning field that had yet to be fully defined and was not always recognized. Employment by women's clubs offered the economic stability necessary for public health nurses to pursue professional recognition of their chosen work.[69]

The backing of prominent clubwomen authorized nurses to undertake many tasks that were beyond the realm of traditional nursing, such as their efforts to provide working-class "patients with lessons in proper middle class health behavior."[70] In Bluefield, West Virginia, for example, the women's club bragged about the ability of its local public health nurse to identify "destitute children" and place them with families.[71] Kentucky clubwomen also worked with public health nurses who had the authority to remove unhealthy children from their homes and transport them to Louisville or Lexington for treatment or surgery.[72]

At times, clubwomen consciously assisted nurses in promoting their professional status. In southwestern Virginia, the Health Committee of the Women's Club of Salem formed the nucleus of the Community Nursing Association, an alliance of public health nurses.[73] The McDowell Women's Club of Welch, West Virginia, enrolled the club on the National Organization of Public Health Nursing's cooperative membership roll.[74]

Female volunteers supported the professional ambitions of young women interested in nursing. West Virginia clubwomen collected donations for a scholarship fund to enable three educated nurses to enroll in special public health training programs. At the same time, the West Virginia federation resolved to promote the introduction of public health nurses into every community and encourage young women to "fit themselves for the public health field."[75]

Such action was championed by the GFWC, whose Division of Health included a Committee on Public Health Nursing. The goal of this committee was to "enlist the active help of clubwomen in demonstrating the public health nurse as an indispensable health servant and securing definite recognition of public health nursing."[76] The GFWC also valued public health nurses as its most important allies in Americanization work, finding them more important than any other social force in modernizing the immigrant's home.[77]

Nurses often served as liaisons between clubwomen and working-class and immigrant families.[78] Clubwomen might have been sincere in their determination to aid those in need of medical service, but they lacked the professional credentials necessary to legitimize their entry into the homes of those targeted for relief.[79] They relied on trained public health nurses, acting as their agents, to undertake that task instead. The GFWC recognized the unique ability of public health nurses, unlike women volunteers, to enter the homes of the disadvantaged as professionals and not providers of charity. The nurse's "services are not considered charity. They are duly paid for, even though slightly, and thus self respect and independence are preserved."[80]

Finally, clubwomen assisted public health nurses in advocating for the legislative and administrative transformations that nurses believed were necessary to advance public welfare. At times, such advocacy was overt. Lucille Price, a physician's wife and clubwoman from Scarbro, West Virginia, made public health a central focus of her legislative work as a member of the House of Delegates.[81] An avid supporter of antituberculosis work, she also promoted maternal and infant health programs.[82] Following a pattern she had developed before women were granted suffrage, she often asked not for votes but for "sympathy and support" for the health reforms she championed.[83]

Price was one of several clubwomen who held political office and used their positions to further the public health ambitions of their colleagues in the voluntary movement. Margaret Kuyk, the chairperson of the Virginia Federation of Women's Clubs' Division of Health in 1923, was employed by the Virginia Department of Public Health.[84] Jean Dillon, a prominent nurse and activist in the West Virginia Department of Public Health, was onetime head of the state's Division of Child Hygiene and Public Health Nursing.[85] She also served as chairperson of the West Virginia Federation of Women's Clubs' Public Health Division.[86] Harriet Jones, a physician, was an enthusiastic clubwoman who was a member of the West Virginia

House of Delegates, a position that enabled her to campaign for public health reform.[87]

Public health nurses and clubwomen had a complicated relationship. Although their social and economic conditions were typically dissimilar, they shared a mutual concern for the well-being of their communities, especially for the health of mothers and children.[88] In more rural communities, nurses labored alongside settlement workers to address the medical needs of the isolated families they targeted for aid. Settlement and Frontier Nursing Service activities had many characteristics in common with the health campaigns undertaken by public health nurses and supported by local women's clubs. These programs, however, were primarily aimed at country people who were uniquely burdened by their isolation from established medical services and their continued reliance on folk healing.

The Frontier Nursing Service, founded in the 1920s by Mary Breckinridge, stands as a unique example of a female-directed and -staffed program intended to bring modern health care to the mountains. Although Breckinridge shared the maternalist concerns that drove many clubwomen and nurses, she was unusual in possessing both a benevolent agenda rooted in her elite class origins and professional credentials as a graduate of a European nurse-midwifery program. Her determination to eradicate lay midwifery, which she considered a danger to women and infants, and to subordinate highly educated nurse-midwives at least nominally to the supervision of physicians illustrates her awareness of the necessity to sacrifice women's potential professional autonomy to achieve improved maternal and infant health.[89]

In 1923, before she established the Frontier Nursing Service, Breckinridge traveled throughout the mountain counties of eastern Kentucky and documented the lack of modern medical care available in the hills. Her report chronicled the practices of lay midwives and denounced the inadequacies of their procedures. Along with these criticisms, Breckinridge lamented the substantial number of physicians who lacked formal training practicing in the mountain counties. These "pseudo-doctors," as she termed them, were "dangerous" and had no "justification whatever for assuming" the title of doctor.[90]

Breckinridge's most disturbing encounter occurred when she met a young couple who, although "clean and intelligent," were "quite the most dangerous of all." The husband, like many nineteenth-

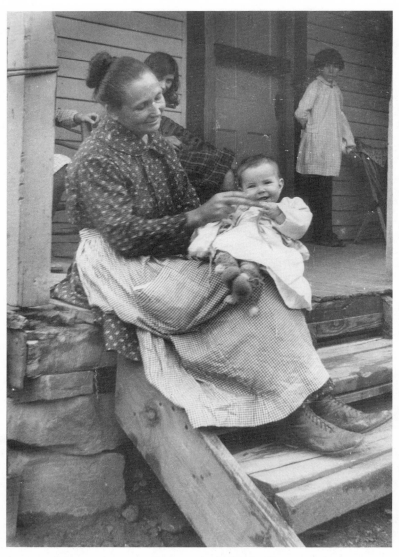

Doctors and women reformers sought to remake the beliefs and practices of mountain mothers like this one from Kentucky. *Audio-Visual Archives, Special Collections and Archives, University of Kentucky Libraries.*

century practitioners, had acquired healing skills through empirical practice and served as the self-proclaimed doctor in an isolated community. His wife was a competent lay midwife, but through her husband and with his authorization, she had acquired a hypodermic needle and sometimes used it to administer pituitrin to hasten labor.

Women, Health Care, and the Community

Her presumption that although she had no formal education she was capable of dispensing medication greatly distressed Breckinridge, who considered the reliance of empirically trained midwives on "pseudo-doctors" to be a "grave problem."[91]

Breckinridge believed that the replacement of traditional healers and midwives with educated nurse-midwives would greatly benefit mountain residents. From the beginning of her work, she sought the aid and guidance of the medical community; many of her outside advisers and financial supporters, in fact, were doctors. Leslie County was selected as the site for the Frontier Nursing Service's pilot program with the guidance and permission of Dr. Arthur T. McCormack, the commissioner of the state board of health, secretary of the state medical alliance, and son of Dr. Joseph N. McCormack, who had made his career crusading for scientific medicine. McCormack approved the selection of Leslie County because no licensed physicians practiced there and thus the Frontier Nursing Service would not be competing with physicians for patients.[92]

Breckinridge continued to court the approval of the Kentucky State Medical Society and the national medical community by constantly involving them in the Frontier Nursing Service's affairs. Two of the nine executive committee positions were held by physicians, as were several of the national board of trustees seats. In addition to these positions, leading doctors from Kentucky and around the nation composed the Frontier Nursing Service's National Medical Council and Medical Advisory Board.[93]

Although the nurse-midwives of the Frontier Nursing Service acted with a great deal of autonomy on a daily basis, the service was nominally subordinate to the dictums of the medical profession. From the beginning, the nurse-midwives sought regular consultations with physicians for troublesome cases and referred extremely difficult cases to hospitals and clinics in Louisville and Lexington. To guide the everyday work of the Frontier Nursing Service's agents, Breckinridge solicited the direction of a number of prominent physicians who compiled a manual of prescribed procedures. This document served as a guide for the nurse-midwives and a constant symbol of their professional subordination to educated physicians.[94]

In spite of the extensive efforts of Breckinridge and her colleagues at other settlement schools, some mountain residents persisted in relying on traditional healers and ignoring the preventive and therapeutic advice of nurses and physicians associated with the settlements. When residents seemed particularly recalcitrant about adopting health care innovations or when the trained professionals at the settlements identified medical needs beyond their ability to handle, additional interventions were offered by settlement workers and their medical allies.[95]

Settlement agents and local public health officials waged campaigns to eradicate the nearly epidemic levels of trachoma, but when their efforts alone were inadequate, they joined forces with men like Dr. J. A. Stucky.[96] Stucky argued that the region's chronic ill health was perpetuated by the absence of legitimate practitioners and by the ignorance of the inhabitants, a position shared by the settlement workers and their middle-class supporters. Stucky and his colleagues offered immediate help to those who placed themselves in his care. His clinic, which provided almost miraculous relief to many trachoma victims, served as exceptionally effective advertising for the promise of scientific medicine. Through such large-scale and impressive projects, physicians and their settlement allies wooed natives to accept the benefits of scientific medicine.[97]

Reformers faced a more difficult challenge when trying to convince pregnant women to embrace the services of educated birth attendants. As we have seen, many of the younger physicians practicing in Appalachia after the turn of the twentieth century were from outside the region and thus did not share the ethnic, geographical, or class identities that enabled rural physicians elsewhere to gradually ease into the birthing rooms as local midwives were exiting.[98] Often unfamiliar with the few physicians who did practice in their counties and wedded to a female-centered model of birth and delivery that was firmly anchored in the community, many Appalachian women saw little reason to reject traditional midwifery in favor of scientific medicine.[99] To encourage them to do so, reformers, male and female, resorted to the use of both the carrot and the stick, enticing women to embrace nurse-midwifery and physician-assisted childbirth as symbols of the advantages of modern life at the same time that they promoted legislation to restrict lay midwives.

The Frontier Nursing Service, which introduced a woman-centered medical model that resembled traditional midwifery more closely than anything else outsiders brought to the mountains, was highly effective in introducing scientific medicine. As a nurse acknowledged in an article in *Southern Mountain Life and Work* in 1925, however, "Old ideas of health change very slowly here."[100] Outsiders

Women, Health Care, and the Community

brought dramatic innovations to the highlands, but these changes were not accepted without resistance and debate.

Opposition to modern medicine emerged because physicians and educated midwives and nurses demanded radical changes in centuries-old traditions. The Frontier Nursing Service, for example, insisted not only that the traditional birth attendant be replaced but also that the very act of giving birth be changed. Breckinridge, in her examination of traditional midwives, noted that it was common practice for women to deliver in an upright position and that mothers were encouraged to walk around to further labor. The dominant expectation among scientific physicians during the 1920s, which Breckinridge appeared to share, was that women should be in a supine position when giving birth. As historians and health care advocates have noted, the horizontal position can actually retard labor and serves only to aid the birth attendant.[101] Walking around also promotes the mother's sense of efficacy and control over her childbirth experience, concerns that scientific medical practitioners did not address.

Mountaineers exhibited a healthy resistance to the imposition of modern practices, choosing instead to carefully select the innovations they wished to employ. Ida Stapleton, a physician with the Pine Mountain Settlement School who worked in the remote settlement at Line Fork, authored a series of fund-raising letters that documented the gradual shift from reliance on traditional care to an appreciation of scientific medicine. Stapleton's letters reveal that Appalachian women demonstrated a shrewd determination to secure the safest, most cost-efficient, and most effective care from their medical providers.

Stapleton, as a trained physician, was unwilling to wait in attendance on a woman nearing her due date, which led to the fear that the doctor would not arrive in time and the patient might deliver with no assistance at all. To avoid this, some women acquired the aid of a "granny" midwife who settled in to assist with the family chores and wait until the delivery occurred.[102]

Other families weighed economic considerations against the type of assistance they needed. Stapleton reported that her services were more expensive than those of midwives but that she offered postnatal care for mothers and infants whereas midwives did not. Midwives, however, often assisted with domestic chores, which physicians did not do.[103] Breckinridge was offended to find that some

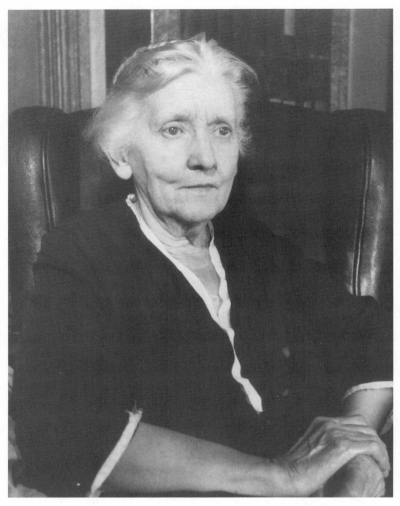

Linda Neville's crusade to regulate midwifery was an extension of her campaign to end blindness. *Audio-Visual Archives, Special Collections and Archives, University of Kentucky Libraries.*

midwives dared to charge $10 for a delivery, the same fee usually required by educated physicians.[104]

Finally, rural families appraised the speed and efficacy of scientific medicine when they judged its value. Stucky's trachoma clinics were beneficial because they offered immediate improvement to the patient. The value of inoculations and vaccinations were increasingly recognized in the 1920s. In less dramatic circumstances, however, families were not always fully convinced of the overwhelming advantage offered by scientific medicine. Stapleton reported that one of her clients chose to use her remedy for thrush rather than a home recipe because the patient "reckoned the doctor's medicine would cure it quicker."[105] Another mountain woman whose child had thrush chose to see a physician because the traditional remedy had not succeeded and so she turned to the settlement doctor for a second opinion.[106]

Although mountain people pursued their own interests when dealing with the medical community, they did not enjoy a free market in which to choose between traditional healers and the innovations of modern medicine. Unlike the empirically trained midwives and traditional doctors native to the region, the settlement workers, clubwomen, and physicians who invaded the mountains were increasingly backed by the weight of the state.[107] Allied with a bureaucracy capable of punishing those who challenged their growing monopoly, modern medical practitioners possessed a clear advantage over their traditional competitors.

The strength of the forces allied against empirically trained healers was evidenced in the campaign by educated physicians and female volunteers to supervise and eventually end the practice of lay midwifery in Appalachia. This alliance was particularly overt in Kentucky, where Linda Neville, a clubwoman and leader of the state antiblindness crusade, allied with the Kentucky State Medical Society to lobby the state legislature to pass laws regulating lay midwifery. Neville was determined to promote the passage of laws requiring that lay midwives be supervised and mandating that preventive measures be taken by midwives to avoid neonatal blindness. To further her plans, Neville wrote to the physicians' lobby asking for aid but acknowledging that physicians' hesitancy to publicly assault midwives was understandable since such an action might be perceived as monopolistic.[108]

Upon receipt of Neville's letter, Dr. Arthur McCormack, the executive secretary of the state medical association and the state commissioner of public health, proposed a solution to his colleagues. Rather than wage the campaign against midwifery themselves, McCormack suggested, the medical association should prepare a bill to regulate midwives and turn it over to Neville and the clubwomen of Kentucky, allowing them to introduce it to members of the legislature. According to McCormack: "We should not appear in the matter, but let it be done by the women . . . [for] if it comes from the women of the state and a demand is made by them that they be protected from these filthy midwives, it would come with great force to our legislators."[109]

Legislation to regulate the practice of midwifery, like laws aimed at supervising the medical profession, gradually eliminated alternative practitioners across Appalachia. Ordered by law to obey the principles of scientific medicine, mountain people also were offered attractive inducements to accept their place as patients in the new medical order.

At the Caney Creek Community Center in eastern Kentucky, local citizens were lured by the possibility of obtaining a "Dream House"—"a three room plank house with windows." Acquisition of this Dream House, according to promotional literature, could be achieved through obedience to the medical authorities of the settlement school, especially to the district nurse, "clean and capable in her white linen uniform." In a fictional account, the nurse, single-handedly and with great finesse and psychological skill, manages to transform a family into clean, obedient, and healthy citizens, who, by the end of the tale, are enthusiastically clamoring for their Dream Home.[110]

Certain conditions had to be met, of course, before an applicant qualified for a Dream Home. Many of the "Requirements for Occupancy of a Dream-Home" were to be expected—"no swearing, no spitting on the floor, no fighting, cursing or shooting." However, listed immediately after these basic demands was the requirement that "all perspective [sic] mothers in the house must submit themselves to the district nurse . . . or to a registered physician, before, during and after childbirth; and all the family must be in the charge of the said nurse, or a registered physician during sickness." These rules were specified before any provisions about either profitable employment or education.[111]

Clubwomen and settlement workers certainly offered the citizens they targeted for assistance important benefits. In addition to the tangible improvements to health provided by scientific medicine, women volunteers proffered social and educational opportunities for rural citizens as well as residents of coal-mining camps through kindergartens, schools, clubs, Americanization classes, cooking exhibits, and sewing and vocational programs. Many Appalachian natives welcomed access to these services, embracing these symbols of twentieth-century life and adjusting quickly to the transformations required of them. Other residents, however, struggled to adapt innovations and therapies to their own will, seeking to avail themselves of new remedies while at the same time trying to guarantee themselves sovereignty over the application of medical knowledge.

By carrying the message of scientific care into mountain villages and mining camps, women volunteers successfully demonstrated the value of their work to educated physicians. As proponents of the medical profession, they proved to be exceptionally efficient allies, recruiting patients and introducing modern medical care to inhabitants of the most remote sections of the region and the poorest mining and timbering settlements.

Their success, however, was often made possible by the low-cost, frequently charitable nature of their work. Women reformers, especially clubwomen, were seldom economic actors accustomed to securing wages for their own work.[112] They were bound to one another and to the medical model through a rhetoric of charity and uplift. United in their benevolent associations, they generally had little motivation or experience to promote the proprietary foundation of medical care that physicians embraced so fervently during the Progressive Era. In fact, many of these activists became strong proponents of the public health movement, pursuing an agenda that potentially questioned the fee-for-service model of health care and challenged the social and economic position enjoyed by private physicians.[113]

As female reformers in clubs and settlement schools gained legitimacy, their enthusiasm over the public health movement became increasingly annoying to private physicians. By the 1920s, women activists and male physicians began to split over the economics of health care. That division contributed to the gradual exodus of many female supporters from the health care discussion and led to the growing reliance of scientifically trained physicians on dependent women's auxiliaries to promote their case before the public.

CHAPTER FIVE

Limiting

Public Health

Appalachian clubwomen and settlement workers, in partnership with public health nurses and guided by physicians, crusaded to ameliorate conditions for women and children in the 1910s and early 1920s. Like their colleagues across the nation, these reformers were part of a cooperative public health movement that enjoyed the support of physicians until doctors, determined to enlarge their domain to include preventive care, began to question the authority of women reformers to speak on medical matters. Both doctors' professional ambitions, revealed in their determination to claim for themselves preventive as well as curative medicine, and the growing conservatism of the 1920s undermined the foundation on which independent women's advocacy for medical practice had been built in Appalachia. These developments ushered in a new era in which the legitimacy of autonomous women's work was degraded and only dependent women directly connected to male physicians were empowered to speak for medical reform.[1]

Although male and female reformers often worked closely together, Maureen Flanagan has demonstrated, fundamental differences defined the presumptions that guided them. Having been raised to fulfill gender-specific expectations, men and women brought different histories and expectations to their alliance in reform campaigns. Like the clubmen Flanagan chronicled in Chicago, doctors spent the majority of their public lives pursuing their professional ambitions and working to achieve economic security. Defined by these experiences, they believed that they improved the lives of poor Appalachians by teaching them how to acquire medical care through the established service model. Clubwomen and settlement workers, however, focused on alleviating the suffering and resolving the disorder that burdened members of their communities, soothing and settling disturbances as mothers would within their households. The nature of the economic model that supported the undertaking was a secondary, if not tertiary, concern.[2]

Many physicians, however, believed that the need to protect and advance the proprietary medical model was a legitimate consequence of their efforts to extend improved health care to Appalachian people. Elite physicians possessed the wealth and standing to support free or low-cost public health programs, but the typical physician who practiced in a coal camp, county seat, or mountain community struggled to encourage the dependence of the local population on his care. When female reformers exhibited a tendency to place the delivery of care above safeguarding the economics of proprietary medicine, physicians began to abandon their previous allies.[3]

Other developments in medical economics exacerbated the reservations physicians were beginning to exhibit about the activities of women reformers. During the 1920s, as the coal economy shrank and opportunities for company doctors declined, nonelite physicians perceived themselves as threatened by expanding public health programs supported by the state. Demanding that public health authorities define their activities in the most narrow terms, doctors challenged what they saw as assaults against their role as caretakers of the community, joining colleagues across the nation in attempting to limit the reach of public health.[4]

Appalachian doctors based their arguments against the expansion of public health in part on developments within the field itself. As Judith Walzer Leavitt and Richard Meckel have argued, by the twentieth century, public health activists had turned from a focus on the community to a fixation on identifying and alleviating public health concerns through attention to the individual. Whether isolating carriers like Typhoid Mary or attempting to alleviate infant and maternal mortality through preventive screenings and education, public health agents redirected their attention from the environment to the individual. As members of the middle class who profited from the exploitation of miners and their families in unsanitary coal camps, mountain physicians welcomed this epistemological shift since it avoided the possibility of criticism of the conditions their friends and neighbors helped create in the coal towns they owned and controlled. The redefinition of the problem of infant mortality as a consequence of maternal illness presented an especially attractive opportunity. By arguing that women's health was key to their children's health, doctors realized that they could expand their private practices into preventive medicine and prophylactic care for pregnant women and infants.[5] To secure that arena, however, they had to remove maternal and infant care from the hands of women reformers and activists.

The low-cost or free nature of public health activities violated the doctors' commitment to the fee-for-service or proprietary model, but physicians were also disturbed by the growing power of female professionals in public health work.[6] As historians Molly Ladd-Taylor, Sheila Rothman, and Theda Skocpol have demonstrated, the attack on the federal Sheppard-Towner Infancy and Maternity Protection Act of 1921 was motivated, in part, by a determination to "rescue public health services from 'lay' women's control."[7] By wresting public health advocacy from the grasp of maternalist reformers, physicians guaranteed both the triumph of the fee-for-service model and their supremacy over female health care providers.

Divisions were not drawn along gender lines alone, however, and female reformers were hardly the passive victims of male physicians. As we will see, female physicians sometimes fought against women reformers to protect the medical profession from challenge by potential competitors. In other cases, middle- and upper-class women advocates allied with doctors against midwives, members of the working class who continued to pose an economic threat to rural Appalachian doctors well into the twentieth century. Growing class divisions, along with the conservatism of the 1920s described by Nancy Cott in *The Grounding of Modern Feminism*, furthered the professional goals of male practitioners at the same time that they undermined the work of independent women's organizations. By the end of the decade, Appalachian women reformers, members of a middle class that had confirmed its standing above the workers who supported the region's economy, sought out and enjoyed fewer opportunities for meaningful health care advocacy as physicians turned their backs on their old allies and increasingly relied on dependent auxiliaries to spread their message.[8]

Dr. J. A. Stucky and his colleagues went to eastern Kentucky to fight trachoma, but they were also seeking to introduce modern medicine and the social and economic systems that accompanied it to the mountaineers. To succeed in this task, doctors required the assistance of settlement workers and other women activists. Dedicated to communicating to Appalachian people the obligations and

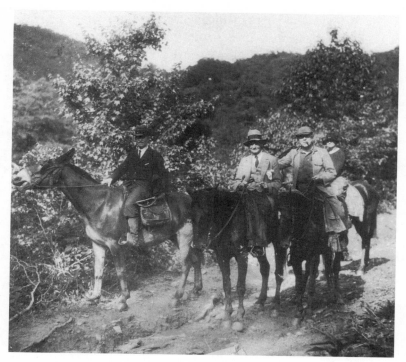

Left to right: Dr. W. J. Hutchins, president of Berea College; Dr. J. A. Stucky, a physician noted for his efforts to eliminate trachoma in eastern Kentucky; and Dr. Arthur T. McCormack, secretary of the Kentucky Board of Health, represented the forces allied to initiate change among mountain residents. Audio-Visual Archives, Special Collections and Archives, University of Kentucky Libraries.

opportunities of industrial life, public health nurses and settlement workers complied with doctors' demands that a fee-for-service philosophy be infused throughout their medical relief programs. Doctors made it clear to philanthropists that they were unwilling to undertake work among the mountaineers as an entirely charitable activity.[9]

Physicians argued that this attitude was not based on thoughtless avarice but that they were actually aiding mountain residents in embracing contemporary life by preventing what Stucky called the "abuse of charity."[10] In a 1911 letter to a nurse at the Hindman Settlement School, he wrote: "Nothing is more fatal to a community than for them to feel they can get services free for which others have to pay. . . . In other words, Miss Butler, make it appear to them a privilege to pay for what they receive."[11]

The women who ran the settlement schools and clinics generally heeded physicians' insistence that they charge for the services they delivered, although they always provided opportunities for poor residents to secure care. At Hindman, an announcement for an eye, ear, nose, and throat clinic proclaimed that "everyone will be expected to pay something for medical service and medicine." It guaranteed that no one would be turned away, however, because of lack of funds and that chickens, eggs, honey, fruit, and baskets would be accepted in trade.[12] The Pine Mountain Settlement School, in its 1934 fund-raising letter, assured subscribers that, "while health work must be of a partly charitable nature," the school disguised this from its clients "in order not to present it to our people as charity."[13] Nurse-midwives at the Frontier Nursing Service proclaimed that "it is not an unusual event to answer a knock at the dispensary door and find one or two very small children who announce, 'We've come to work for you all to get our dipthery.'"[14] By inculcating the youngsters with the message of proprietary medicine, the settlements prepared them for their roles in the larger commercial economy.

In the mountains, doctors sought to introduce and affirm the proprietary system of modern medical delivery at the same time that they inaugurated widespread campaigns to bring the benefits of trained care to rural communities. By linking the fee-for-service model with access to educated practitioners, doctors attempted to confirm in the countryside the traditions that were gaining legitimacy in towns across the United States.

In order to promote the fee-for-service model, physicians had to negotiate with settlement workers and clubwomen, whose maternalist sentiments legitimized their claim to speak as defenders of mothers and children. These women confidently asserted their right to foster public health reform.[15] Vera Harvey, president of the West Virginia Federation of Women's Clubs, demanded recognition of the importance of women's judgment about matters related to "food, health, and the care and education of children." She proclaimed that "the advice of sensible women about these matters will be much better for the country than propaganda of press agents and lobbyists hired to . . . profit some private interest."[16] Women activists did not publicly acknowledge their awareness of the inconsistency of their allegiance to physicians who were themselves a "private interest" seeking to manipulate public events to their advantage through health campaigns.

Appalachian physicians gradually came to oppose the independence of women reformers because they challenged the developing presumption that doctors were the sole authorities over preventive as well as curative health care.[17] This ideal gained ground in the 1920s and was discussed frequently in the region's medical publications. To promote the intellectual shift required as doctors moved beyond curative medicine and into preventive care, physicians used their medical journals to encourage one another to assume responsibility for the continued well-being of their patients as well as for curing them when they were ill. In the *Virginia Health Bulletin*, mountain doctors joined their colleagues from other parts of the state in insisting that citizens recognize that constant obedience to a doctor's commands was the sole road to sustained good health. An article entitled "Health Insurance—The Real Kind" informed readers that compliance with a doctor's orders was the only legitimate health insurance.[18]

In "Agencies That Would Clip the Wings of Medical Progress," a presentation delivered at the 1925 West Virginia State Medical Association meeting in Bluefield, Harry Hall lauded doctors for their persistent efforts to fight disease and their ongoing battle to find new remedies or preventions for contagious illnesses. Hall reminded his audience, however, that although these endeavors aided the general population, they were not necessarily beneficial to the interests of private doctors.[19]

Hall argued that "it would be good business for a doctor to let Typhoid Germs swarm by the trillions. It would be good hard headed commercialism for doctors not to vaccinate." He proclaimed that doctors nevertheless continued to contribute to the public health of the community in spite of the negative consequences of such actions on their own incomes. Although Hall's tirade was extreme, he was not alone in his concern over the competition private physicians faced from programs aimed at improving public health.[20]

Like Hall and his colleagues in Appalachia, physicians throughout the United States reexamined their attitudes toward public health during the 1920s. Throughout most of the Progressive Era, physicians promoted reforms that improved the health of citizens across the nation and the Appalachian region. These efforts also served the doctors' interests by solidifying their professional hegemony and denying legitimacy to alternative practitioners. By the 1920s, as Ronald Numbers has documented in his classic work on health insurance, many doctors, especially those loyal to the American Medical Association (AMA), came to fear the progressive trends exhibited by the government and voluntary organizations.[21]

In a defense of country doctors, W. W. Kerns, a general practitioner engaged in rural practice, argued that public health units undercut private physicians by offering services at lower costs than those of private doctors. "In steps the State with the County Health Unit to take a whack at us," he wrote, "vaccinating children and everyone else for 10 cents, for which we get $1.00, using toxin-antitoxin for 50 cents for which we get $3.00, using typhoid fever antitoxin from 60 cents to $1.00 for which we get $5.00, holding tonsil clinics and charging $10.00 for half doing the job."[22]

Kerns also belittled the supervisory responsibilities of local public health agents who were empowered to enforce state laws requiring that doctors submit full and accurate accounts of the births and deaths they attended. The administrative authority of the local public health officers particularly annoyed Kerns since, unlike physicians in private practice, public health agents were seldom required to respond to emergencies. "How about the county health physicians?," asked Kerns. "Do they get up at midnight, drive eight to ten miles to relieve the suffering of some poor woman or child? Not by a long shot."[23]

The campaign by Monongalia County, West Virginia, physicians to obstruct the establishment of a public health unit in their county illustrates the opposition of doctors to what they perceived to be the competition inherent in the creation of a government-funded public health office. Although it occurred in the northern coalfields of West Virginia, the Monongalia County doctors' resistance provides us with some understanding of the challenges faced by advocates of public health programs in Central Appalachia during the early twentieth century.

The first Board of Health of the State of West Virginia was created by the legislature in 1881. Although the state began to move toward modern standards of sanitation and hygiene in the nineteenth century, each county was left to choose whether or not it wanted to create a public health unit. Throughout the first decades of the twentieth century, counties across the state began establishing city, county, consolidated city-county, or regional health units.[24]

Lacking aggressive leadership from the local medical society, Monongalia County was slow to build a public health system. The medical association had not been particularly sympathetic to the idea of the creation of a county public health unit, but it had never actively opposed it. By 1929, however, new agitation for a public health office met with open resistance from the county's doctors.[25] Rather than continue their benign neglect, the members of the Monongalia County Medical Society expressed a growing fear of socialism and state intervention that was shared by many of their colleagues throughout the region. These fears were so strong that several county medical associations beseeched the West Virginia attorney general to investigate "Socialized Medicine."[26]

As the physicians struggled with their concerns over methods of payment and government interference in their profession, the community was becoming increasingly adamant in its demand for a county public health unit. In 1927, nearly 1,000 rural residents, many of whom lived in the coal camps along Scotts Run, petitioned the county court to establish a public health office. When those pleas were ignored, more than 1,200 citizens signed a similar petition the next year.[27] In spite of the support of these rural citizens, the court did not take the issue under advisement until the summer of 1929, when a visiting physician convinced the local newspaper editor and the members of the county court of the value of such an agency. He received, however, a less enthusiastic response from many local doctors.[28]

Following a speech by this public health advocate, the members of the county medical society retired to discuss the merits of a public health office for the county. In their meeting, they debated the usefulness of free inoculations and warned of the dangers of "state medicine." After much disagreement, the doctors consented to accept the formation of a county health department if it did not actually practice curative medicine. As long as its duties were limited to inoculations and sanitation issues, they agreed not to actively oppose the measure when it came before the county court.[29]

The medical community was primarily concerned with the issue of payment and the danger of government intervention between the physician and his client. The society's legislative committee revealed its apprehension over potential competition from the public health unit when it insisted that patients who were able to afford medical or surgical treatment be referred to private physicians because "we feel it is unfair to the taxpayers of the county to bear the expense of medical and surgical services to those who are able to pay for the same, nor, do we feel it is just to the medical profession that such people be treated by the Board of Health or other agency of like character."[30]

In the two weeks before the county court voted on the issue, supporters of the public health unit brought strong pressure against the ambivalent physicians. An editorial in the *New Dominion* pointed out that few doctors practiced in Monongalia County outside the county seat of Morgantown, arguing that the health of citizens in "the thickly populated mining sections" should not "be sacrificed because public immunizations against contagions and infections can be given free."[31] The newspaper also reminded its readers that 40 percent of the annual budget of the public health unit would be paid by grants from the state and federal governments and the Rockefeller Foundation.[32]

Despite these practical advantages, Morgantown's physicians would not condone the creation of an institution founded on the principles of "social medicine." At the county court session convened to decide the matter, some of the city's doctors sought to postpone the vote. They were defeated, however, and the county court, over the opposition of many physicians, voted to raise the money to establish a public health unit.[33]

Besides opposing propositions that used government funds to finance medical services that might compete with proprietary health care delivery, private physicians also opposed public health campaigns administered by private associations. They were discomforted by the economic structures that supported public health programs, but they also came to reject the active involvement of lay organizations in this work. Unlike physicians who promulgated inoculation campaigns or advocated improved sanitation as a demonstration of their benevolence, lay advocates who organized public health programs crossed accepted boundaries and challenged the professional domination of medical practice by daring to speak about both the content of medicine and the delivery of care.[34] Their work undermined the social and economic monopoly physicians sought and threatened doctors' assertions that health care was a privilege to be purchased in the private market, not a right to be acquired through public funds.

Initially, physicians applauded the health programs established by settlement workers and clubwomen because many rural Appalachian citizens simply did not know when to seek or how to acquire the services of private practitioners without their aid. Although doctors were often unwilling to set up practices in impoverished rural communities, they recognized the needs of isolated citizens and acknowledged that as long as private physicians would not locate in the countryside, public health agents had a legitimate mission. In a letter to the *Virginia Medical Monthly*, Dr. Charles Webb argued that the continued high mortality from typhoid in rural communities "may be the fault of the medical profession," which had failed to appropriately vaccinate and care for potential victims.[35] His concern was legitimized by statistics from the Virginia Board of Health, which documented low rates of diphtheria immunization in Appalachian counties of the state and accordingly high rates of infection and death.[36]

Lacking private physicians in their communities, the *Virginia Medical Monthly* commented, rural citizens turned to traditional healers and "quacks and fakirs." To prevent their reliance on these unacceptable practitioners, educated doctors, allied with their state and local boards of health, realized that the government had to step in to provide minimum health benefits for rural citizens. These programs, however, were to be limited and were at all costs to be under the control of the various state medical associations and state boards of health. As a representative of the Virginia Board of Health stated in 1927: "Our policy is to help the public, but our policy is not to hurt the doctor; on the contrary, it is to help the doctor."[37]

One way to help doctors was to prevent nonprofessional volunteer groups from implementing public health programs without medical supervision or involvement. In a 1927 article entitled "Doctors Disapprove Children's Clinic," a Virginia newspaper reported that physicians in southwestern Virginia's medical societies opposed the activities of outsiders who initiated clinics for disabled children. These programs, supported by women's clubs and held with the cooperation of the state orthopedist, provided free or low-cost care to the children of the area. Local doctors resisted this practice, however, because they felt it undermined their role in the community and limited the number of orthopedic cases treated by resident physicians. Although they opposed these clinics, the members of the medical society assured the female volunteers that "the movement was not intended to deprecate the work of the Woman's Club."[38]

Other Virginia physicians were less considerate of the work initiated by female volunteers. Describing women's public health activities, an officer of the Virginia State Medical Society who also held a position with the state Department of Health wrote that "charitable people put up a lot of money and, being all dressed up with nowhere to go, put on clinics. The women some time ago became obsessed with the idea of clinics; they wanted every child diagnosed and cured in those clinics." He reassured his colleagues in the medical society that the Department of Health would not do any curative work and that it was turning child welfare and antituberculosis work over to local chapters of the medical society as quickly as possible.[39]

Doctors' desire to control charitable work was particularly obvious after the start of the Great Depression. In 1931, the Virginia State Medical Society published a protocol for managing charitable endeavors in which it asserted that county medical societies should have the authority to investigate benevolent health care activities and judge each program's worthiness. The quantity of free medical and hospital care should be examined by local medical associations to determine "if the charity work extended is out of proportion to the needs of the local community."[40]

Physicians questioned the funding of public health programs in both rural communities and settled towns in the 1920s. In an advertisement for a clinic at Big Creek in Clay County, Kentucky, Dr. C. B. Marcum and Linda Neville, the founder of the Mountain Fund, addressed such concerns by offering a lengthy defense of the financing of their public health screenings. According to their promotional literature, at the previous year's clinic, a number of people had erroneously believed that the project was conducted by "the Government or by some agency or other." Acting under that assumption, many patients who could have afforded payment failed to contribute to the operation's coffers. To prevent a similar occurrence this year, the poster clearly informed potential patients of the financial obligations they incurred when receiving care.[41]

Government and private groups that sought to initiate public health campaigns followed Marcum and Neville's model and responded to physicians' opposition by limiting projects to avoid challenging the sanctity of proprietary medical practice. To placate independent physicians, public and private supporters of preventive health work circumscribed their activities and attempted to negotiate acceptable limits for public health ventures, a process similar to the negotiations that Judith Walzer Leavitt has recorded between physicians and public health officials in Milwaukee.[42] The parameters they imposed on preventive care demonstrated the supremacy of proprietary medicine. Public health advocates recognized that it was sometimes necessary to sacrifice the immediate interests of their

Limiting Public Health

targeted populations in order to ensure the general tolerance of the private medical community toward their work.

At the state level, private physicians used their organized strength to resist the extension of government-supported public health practice across Appalachia. Members of the Kentucky State Medical Society insisted that any "full-time health department that fails to increase the office practice of every physician in the county . . . is a failure" since one of the health department's "main objectives is to teach their people the necessity for the use of scientific medicine."[43]

Individual programs were often targeted by physicians, and their activities were curtailed to prevent conflict. Dr. Ennion G. Williams, the health commissioner of Virginia, wrote a public letter to the members of the Otolaryngological and Ophthalmological Society of Virginia in 1929 defending the state's inspection of mountain schoolchildren to identify nose and throat ailments. Williams assured private physicians that the state would limit its involvement to inspection and referral to family doctors, insisting that it would provide no therapeutic services. For the government to offer curative assistance or in any way interfere in the economic relationship between patient and physician would, he asserted, be "State Medicine, something all of us wish to avoid."[44]

To avoid accusations that they were practicing state medicine, public health officers frequently denied their patients anything beyond the most minimal treatment. In the fall of 1927, the health officer of Logan County, West Virginia, examined the schoolchildren of the Island Creek coal district and discovered that 28 percent of them suffered from malnutrition and were more than 10 percent underweight. To remedy this situation, Dr. P. B. Wingfield, the county public health officer, asked the Island Creek Company to furnish cod liver oil and tomato juice to improve the children's diets. No additional medical measures were taken to remedy the children's situation; they were, of course, referred to their "family physicians" for further care.[45] When the president of the West Virginia State Medical Association held a free clinic in Mingo County, West Virginia, in 1930, he was careful to examine only patients who were publicly identified as indigent. Even then, "the persons needing treatment were referred to their family physician and a report of the findings was sent to the physicians interested."[46]

Doctors sometimes resisted public health initiatives with such vigor that public health advocates were driven to express their frustration with individual doctors. Harriet Butler, the first public health nurse at the Hindman Settlement School in Kentucky, wrote to Dr. Joseph N. McCormack, the secretary of the state board of health, in 1911 to protest the opposition of county physicians to her efforts. She recounted the resistance local doctors had demonstrated to her plan to immunize residents against a recent outbreak of diphtheria. Some doctors refused to visit those who were ill with the disease; one physician informed Butler that he thought it "unnecessary to expose himself."[47]

Butler insisted that her intent was "to increase the respect and confidence of the people for the physicians." "But," she added, "some times it is hard." She also assured McCormack that she recognized the concerns of the private physicians and that she had done her utmost to consider their interests as she went about her public health work. "We are trying," she wrote, "to get the clinic started on the right basis having people pay according as they are able."[48] Her protest, qualified by the appropriate reservations, expressed the frustration of public health workers who found their work stymied by an unsympathetic private medical community.

But settlement workers and government health agents refused to completely abandon preventive and educational programs. As they worked together to further these programs, female government workers, public health nurses, and women advocates developed rich networks that led private physicians to become increasingly suspicious. As the debate over Sheppard-Towner projects in Appalachia reveals, private physicians eventually moved to limit the boundaries of public health as well as the parameters of acceptable nonprofessional involvement in advocating and financing medical care.

The medical profession opposed the Sheppard-Towner Act for a number of reasons. Along with their refusal to acknowledge the existence of a crisis in maternal and infant welfare, some doctors articulated their distrust of government intervention in medical care. Of equal or even greater concern to many physicians, however, was the increased autonomy the act secured for public health nurses and other health care advisers and educators.[49]

Medical practitioners, committed to protecting their fledgling claim to sole authority over childbirth, were unwilling to accept the personal sovereignty implied by many of the educational programs offered through Sheppard-Towner. In an era when doctors increasingly resorted to interventionist strategies to hasten labor and promoted the hospital as the only acceptable place to give birth, physicians were adamantly opposed to programs that encouraged independence in childbearing women.

Advertisements in medical journals of the day catered to the physician's belief that he alone was capable of providing accurate information to mothers about their own health and the health of their infants.[50] In promotions for its infant formulas published in medical journals in Appalachia and across the nation, Mead Johnson and Company, a national pharmaceutical enterprise, assured doctors that "Mead's Infant Diet Materials are advertised only to physicians. No feeding directions accompany trade packages."[51] A later advertisement promised Virginia doctors that "we refer patients to physicians at every opportunity."[52]

Parke, Davis and Company, a pharmaceutical corporation that billed itself as the largest in the world in 1931, circulated advertisements that glorified physicians while vilifying traditional healers. A blurb for digitalis portrayed an elderly female herbalist who sold her secret potion for "the clink of golden sovereigns." Having acquired the recipe, an educated male physician experimented with it and created a "new and powerful drug." In the hands of Parke, Davis and Company, the herb was standardized and transformed into a pharmaceutical product.[53]

Physicians, as these advertisements suggest, were moving toward an increasingly professional model of care that recognized them as the sole arbiters of medical diagnosis, prevention, and intervention. At the same time, however, nurses and their allies were reaping the professional and social bounties of the unique opportunities created by the Sheppard-Towner Act. From their position outside the doctor's professional realm, female advocates and their allies in nursing promulgated policies and initiated reforms that potentially challenged doctors' authority.[54]

The battle over midwifery stands as a singular example of the contest between female reformers and more conservative medical practitioners. Although some activists such as Linda Neville enthusiastically supported efforts by the medical community to eradicate traditional midwifery, other volunteers and public health nurses promoted a more balanced perspective that advocated the education and supervision of lay midwives and tolerance of their continued service in rural areas.

Physicians who were struggling to rid themselves of lay midwives and transform childbirth into a medical process found such a view

to be anathema to their professional ambitions. Their desire to eliminate the practice of midwifery was based on their sincere belief that
the care they promised parturient women was superior to anything
mothers might receive from empirically trained midwives.[55] As an
examination of the medicalization of childbirth in rural Canada
during this same era reveals, however, doctors were also threatened
by competition from the growing number of healers entering the
health care marketplace. As campaigns against sectarians and competition between general practitioners and specialists occurred in
the professional arena, physicians also worried about rivalry from
midwives.[56] Their fears were fostered by comments from progressive maternalists like Children's Bureau director Julia Lathrop, who
claimed that "the attention of a poor physician is more dangerous
than that of a good midwife." For liberal activists like Lathrop, the
quality of care, not the professional status of the caregiver, was the
critical issue.[57]

Inevitably, doctors stridently resisted the potential elevation of
midwives through formal education and legal recognition. The
Southern Medical Journal, the publication of the regional medical association, whose members included many Appalachian physicians,
featured a number of articles that addressed "the midwife problem."
E. R. Hardin, a doctor from North Carolina, challenged the education and elevation of lay midwives by asserting that "it gives the
midwife a professional status and establishes two standards where
there should be but one."[58] Walter Edmond Levy, another physician,
rejected the idea of educating lay midwives and argued for "effec-
tively obliterating the midwife, our medical menace."[59]

The author of an editorial in the West Virginia Medical Journal in 1926
harshly criticized a bill authorizing the training and licensing of
midwives. The bill had passed in 1925, according to the editorial,
because the medical association had been preoccupied with the
"hubbub" over the legislative fight to prevent the licensing of chiropractors. The midwife bill, the writer argued, had been a mistake
from the beginning, and the state commissioner of health, who was
closely allied with the West Virginia State Medical Association, was
"thoroughly disgusted with its operation."[60]

In addition to their opposition to educating lay midwives, doctors feared the potential for competition that might emerge if the
nurse-midwifery model promoted by the Frontier Nursing Service
became popular. Although doctors tolerated, and often encouraged,
the activities of the Frontier Nursing Service in rural areas of east-

ern Kentucky, they did not embrace such activities in more urban communities.

The paucity of doctors in the mountains of eastern Kentucky, coupled with Mary Breckinridge's social position, convinced the medical community to accept and even assist her project as a novelty that did not threaten their economic position. In spite of their general acquiescence, however, doctors expressed occasional, and sometimes powerful, opposition to her ambitious project.[61]

Nancy Schrom Dye has documented that when Breckinridge initially sought support from the Commonwealth Fund, a national philanthropy, her efforts were stymied by Dr. Annie Veech, who headed the Kentucky Bureau of Maternal and Child Health. Veech rejected Breckinridge's plans for two reasons. Like many female reformers who worked on Sheppard-Towner projects, Veech insisted that educating lay midwives was the most reasonable and economical way to meet the immediate needs of Kentucky's rural mothers. Breckinridge believed that reliance on formally educated, highly skilled nurse-midwives, supported by physicians when necessary, was the only way to lower the region's high infant and maternal mortality rates. Veech, however, held that empirically trained local women were capable of learning the necessary precautions and improving their skills to a level that would allow them to practice with some autonomy under the supervision of trained medical professionals. Traditional midwives were not an ideal or permanent solution, however; the objective standard, according to Veech, was the physician who alone was capable of providing acceptable care. Veech was willing to continue to tolerate lay midwives in rural communities or among minority populations because they would, in her opinion, eventually vanish in the face of improving standards of medical care. Inherent in this argument was Veech's rejection of the professional status demanded by nurse-midwives. Like many doctors, she was determined to ensure that nurses remain subordinate and maintain their ancillary position in the medical hierarchy.[62]

If doctors rejected the concept of educating lay midwives and elevating nurse-midwives to a professional level, they were equally wary of the increased autonomy of public health nurses. Jane Ransom, the director of Virginia's Bureau of Public Health Nursing, wrote in 1919 that "it has been practically demonstrated that public health nurses are the natural 'answer' to the various needs in the public health field." Her statement contradicted doctors' assertions of their central role in public health, but it reflected an opinion that, according to Barbara Melosh, was common among public health nurses across the country at the time.[63]

The increased authority and freedom public health nurses enjoyed as they staffed and administered the many new programs funded by the Sheppard-Towner Act nourished doctors' mistrust of their actions. As independent field nurses, public health educators, and school inspectors, these women gained legitimacy and furthered their professional maturity. Empowered by these advances, nurses sometimes opposed doctors and resisted policies they believed were detrimental to their patients.

This new strength was fostered by the close relations that developed between administrators of the Children's Bureau, the federal agency responsible for distributing Sheppard-Towner funds, and public health nurses at the state level. Without such mutual support, women leaders would have had little success in moving their reform agendas forward.[64] In West Virginia, for example, Jean Dillon, head of the Division of Child Hygiene and Public Health Nursing during the 1920s, was an intimate friend of Dr. Blanche Haines, the director of the Division of Maternity and Infant Hygiene at the Children's Bureau. The two frequently mixed business with pleasure when Haines came to West Virginia to tour Sheppard-Towner programs, and their correspondence reflects the depth of affection they shared for each other.[65]

Dillon's letters also reveal something of the frustration she and her colleagues experienced as they fought to accomplish their mission in the face of resistance from the often inflexible medical community. One of Dillon's missives to Haines related the story of a doctor who was outraged at the repercussions of the state's Motherhood Correspondence Course, designed by Dillon's office to educate rural mothers about pregnancy and childbirth. The physician in question insisted, "That D——d Motherhood Correspondence Course has got to stop! I can't even go to church anymore without some woman handing me a bottle of urine." This was a consequence of the course's instructions that pregnant women have a urinalysis test done by a physician as a routine part of their prenatal care. The nurses informed the doctor that his predicament was a demonstration of the success of the program and that the correspondence course would continue.[66]

This story offers amusing insight into the conflicts that perturbed public health nurses, but other accounts reveal deeper dissension between nurses and doctors. Red Cross visitors reported that when they attempted to talk with Dr. Henshaw, the director of the West Virginia Department of Health, he gave them a polite interview but expressed little or no interest in maternal and infant welfare. When asked a question about a specific maternal health care program, the Red Cross agent claimed, Henshaw "didn't look as if he had thought of it lately."[67] Dillon, whose division was under the administration of the Department of Health, found the climate there so frustrating that she reported to another Red Cross visitor that "she did not know whom she could trust."[68]

Public health nurses, by the very nature of their professional definitions and ambitions, were both unwilling and unable to accept the absolute authority of the medical community.[69] Mary Ritter Beard, a leader of the national public health movement of the Progressive Era, reminded readers of her instructive texts that public health nurses were often forced on communities by organizations like women's clubs. To earn the respect of the clients they sought to assist, nurses first had to prove that the services they offered were of value.[70] Public health nurses, therefore, had to be assertive, competent, and highly independent as they responded to the complicated situations they encountered every day.

Medical doctors frequently denied public health nurses the respect or recognition their professional behavior demanded. Indeed, many doctors feared the presence of public health nurses and distrusted the premises on which public health education was based. Nurses, Barbara Melosh and Susan Reverby have convincingly argued, were an emerging professional class, and their ambitions and abilities threatened the monopoly over health care enjoyed by physicians.[71] As Karen Buhler-Wilkerson has documented in her study of public health nurses, alliances with voluntary associations temporarily enhanced the legitimacy of public health nursing, but they provided only a flimsy foundation for the elevation of nurses' professional status. When nurses moved into government employment in the 1920s and 1930s, they had few ties to support their efforts to expand their professional capital and were often resented by male physicians for their traditions of independence and their image as an elite nursing corps.[72]

Conflicts between Appalachian doctors and nurses were legion. David Littlejohn, acting commissioner of the West Virginia Department of Public Health during the 1930s, wrote to a colleague at the U.S. Public Health Service that he did not think nurses should be allowed to provide examinations and tuberculosis tests for schoolchildren, arguing that such work was better left to a family physician.[73] The Monongalia County Medical Society of northern West Virginia expressed its attitude toward the county's newly hired public health nurse more blatantly. In 1921, the society commented that she was acceptable only because "she did not pose as one whose knowledge was superior to the doctors."[74]

Nurses who openly challenged doctors suffered professional retribution. Jean Dillon's career as a reformer in a myriad of public health efforts proves the price outspoken professional nurses had to pay if they contradicted the established medical hierarchy. Dillon, a college-educated woman, was both a trained nurse and a former journalist.[75] Professionally, she was active in the state nurses' association and during the 1920s served in the Department of Public Health as director of the Division of Child Hygiene, overseeing Sheppard-Towner programs. She was also an active member and officer of the West Virginia Federation of Women's Clubs and various other benevolent organizations.[76] Throughout her career, Dillon battled medical men who distrusted her professional competence and ambition. Although engaged in the volunteer movement, Dillon devoted only a portion of her abundant energies to the cause. She served on committees for the West Virginia Federation of Women's Clubs and the antituberculosis leagues, but she published few reports for those groups and seldom acted as a major figure in their work.[77] Her voluntary efforts were subordinate to her career, but through her employment, she actively promoted policies to improve the conditions of Appalachian women and children, a campaign that led her into conflict with physicians who insisted on absolute obedience from nurses and other underlings.

Dillon expressed her frustration with medical practitioners in a speech she gave at the 1924 convention of the West Virginia State Nurses' Association. In her discussion of the importance of public health nurses in antituberculosis and maternal and infant care work, she defended the role of public education and challenged the physicians' argument that they should be the central figures in any program related to health care. "We no longer look upon the man of medicine as a man of mystery," she asserted.[78] Dillon did not limit her candor to female audiences. She was equally intrepid in her actions as head of the Division of Child Hygiene. Visitors from the national Red Cross office commented on her willingness to speak "freely and frankly" and on the constant opposition she met from male physicians.[79]

Limiting Public Health

Dillon's lengthy battles with physicians culminated in what was perhaps the inevitable outcome. During the late 1920s, the West Virginia State Medical Association waged a successful campaign demanding that medical doctors head the various divisions of the Department of Health. Dillon did not satisfy this criterion and was removed from her post. Contemporary observers believed that the policy was initiated with the intention of terminating Dillon's employment.[80]

Physicians recognized that the actions of individual nurses such as Dillon were merely symptoms of the growing independence of the nursing profession and attempted to fundamentally alter the institutions that spawned these potential rivals. Joining their colleagues throughout the nation, physicians in Virginia, Kentucky, and West Virginia moved to seize control of their state boards of nursing and assert increased authority over the processes by which they licensed nurses. These initiatives were not open assaults on the public health movement, but they occurred during the same period that nurses were acquiring increased professional status through public health programs.

Campaigns to limit the authority of nurses were not unique to Appalachia in this era, according to Reverby and Melosh. In Ordered to Care, Reverby relates the story of a physician in the 1890s who proposed that in exchange for free lodging nurses work without pay, motivated to do so by their maternal and domestic urges. Such absurd notions were quickly dismissed, but in the 1920s, physicians across the country were still railing against any suggestion that nurses were colleagues or coworkers of doctors. The struggle between nurses and physicians over professionalization in Appalachia is revealed through an examination of nurses' efforts to elevate training standards as a way to improve their professional credentials. Like physicians, nurses sought to solidify their specialized knowledge, improve their educational facilities, and collaborate with the state to formalize their professional authority. As Reverby argues, physicians and hospital administrators across the United States resisted such efforts, just as they did in Appalachia.[81]

The Weather Vane, the journal of the West Virginia State Nurses' Association, published an article in September 1929 celebrating the defeat of a bill sponsored by physicians to restructure the West Virginia Nursing Licensure Board. The bill proposed giving doctors an equal number of seats on the board, denying nurses the power to make policy without the doctors' approval. During the debate over the bill, a nurse offered the following anonymous plea: "[The doctor] has given us paternal interest and has taught us to walk alone, but he is loathe to let go our hand and let us stand alone. We are grateful to the Doctor for his support and his teachings and we need to work together always, but we have passed the stages of babyhood, childhood and adolescence in nursing procedure and we have reached womanhood, with knowledge, responsibility and independence."[82]

Similar efforts were initiated in other Appalachian states. Virginia's nurses faced a strikingly analogous predicament seven years later when a doctor in the state legislature introduced a bill that gave physicians control of the board that licensed nurses. To resist this move, Frances Helen Zeigler, the president of the Graduate Nurses' Association of Virginia, took to the radio waves to arouse public opposition to the bill. In her radio address, Zeigler accused practitioners who sought a place on the state board of nurse examiners of being driven by a desire to reduce the professional status and authority of nurses.[83]

Zeigler's evaluation of the situation was fundamentally accurate. Dr. William Woodson, the state senator who introduced the bill, was the physician in charge of the Piedmont Sanitorium, a state-supported tuberculosis refuge that also trained nurses. Woodson, like many doctors affiliated with nurses' training hospitals, was frustrated by the rising standards that the nursing board imposed on such institutions. Many smaller hospitals, especially proprietary facilities operated by local physicians, were endangered by the tougher requirements their students had to satisfy before they would be accepted by the nursing examiners. To thwart the trend toward rising professional standards among nurses and ensure the continuation of the overproduction of graduates that kept wages low, Woodson and his allies sought to alter the composition of the board and reduce the autonomy and training of educated nurses. As in West Virginia, the effort was unsuccessful, although in Virginia the nurses won in the legislature by only one vote.[84]

During their struggles to limit the parameters of public health and circumscribe the role of government in health care delivery, doctors gradually grew more uncomfortable with the continued involvement of autonomous voluntary organizations in dispensing medical service. Faced with nurses' growing professional status and frightened by the potential competition inherent in the state-funded public health system, physicians gradually came to oppose the autonomy of women volunteers and settlement workers. These former allies had proven themselves to be more independent than doctors had anticipated.

The physicians' gradual rejection of autonomous women's groups was not unique to Appalachia. As historians have documented, the 1920s were marked by conservatism and the ultimate rejection of maternalist principles. As women succumbed to a growing consumer culture that promoted personal gratification over social reform and discouraged intimate female relations as abnormal, they increasingly retreated from public reform activity grounded in gender-specific concerns.[85]

In West Virginia, growing class divisions and intensified labor antagonism during the 1920s shaped women's public activities. Although they were willing to address the immediate health care needs of working-class families, clubwomen were increasingly less willing to contemplate the social or economic forces that created those needs. When, for example, the members of the Virginia Federation of Women's Clubs considered the need for public health nurses to aid poor, rural women, they acknowledged that it was unfair that they had easy access to medical care while other women did without, but their only response was to debate the possibility of imposing a tax on cosmetics to fund public health efforts. In their bulletin, they inquired, "Is it asking too much of the women of Virginia to contribute through this tax a small percent of what they spend in luxuries toward defraying the expenses of health work which will bring relief to the less fortunate women and children?"[86]

In a 1919 report, a chairperson of the Department of Public Health of the West Virginia Federation of Women's Clubs reminded her readers that poor nutrition was not just a problem of the impoverished but that middle- and upper-class children also suffered from malnutrition. She encouraged her colleagues to consider the needs of all children and not to spend a disproportionate amount of time attending to the distress of the poor.[87]

In Williamson, West Virginia, the local newspaper reported that instances of disease were exceptionally high during the winter of 1920. The rate of infectious illness rose, in part, because of the unsanitary conditions prevalent in the tent colonies occupied by striking miners and their families. Local women's clubs and the Red Cross left assistance for the miners to outside agencies but proudly announced that they had raised $5,000 for European relief efforts.[88]

Clubwomen displayed their most blatant commitment to the status quo in their response to the miners' uprising that occurred in southern West Virginia in the summer of 1921. Frustrated by harsh working conditions and the denial of their civil liberties, miners revolted in an effort to open the Mingo County coalfields to union organizers. This crisis, which has been well documented by Appalachian historians, demonstrated the tremendous gulf that separated miners from more affluent coal operators and professionals.[89]

Although members of the West Virginia Federation of Women's Clubs were generally silent about the events that culminated in the battle of Blair Mountain, where thousands of prounion forces clashed with agents loyal to Logan County sheriff Don Chafin and to the coal operators who supported his regime, they did make an official statement at their annual convention in 1922. The clubwomen expressed their displeasure over the events of the previous summer in a resolution that defined their interpretation of the conflict between miners and coal operators and their government allies. They stated: "Open hostility to organized government . . . by radicals who desire the overthrow of constitutional government and the destruction of organized society, and their flagrant circulation of malicious propaganda directed against American ideals and American institutions, has resulted in inciting several thousand men to insurrection against the government of West Virginia and the government of the United States."[90]

The clubwomen expressed their regret over the lives lost at Blair Mountain but verbalized a class-appropriate anger that "these radical leaders have caused the fair name of West Virginia to be maligned."[91] Like the middle-class women who objected to exposés documenting the labor practices that produced working-class poverty, West Virginia's clubwomen were more alarmed by the potential public relations damage than they were by the events themselves.[92]

Periodically, other Appalachian women's clubs denounced organized labor throughout the 1920s. The Tazewell Women's Club in southwestern Virginia, for example, sent several telegrams to the White House expressing its displeasure over the ambitions and policies of organized labor in the coalfields.[93]

The growing conservatism of Appalachian clubwomen in the 1920s can be seen in their affiliation with the American Constitutional Association, an antilabor group founded in West Virginia in response to workers' unrest in 1919 and 1920. Established to deter the spread of the United Mine Workers of America into the coalfields of Central Appalachia, the American Constitutional Association spouted a mixture of nativist, antilabor, and probusiness sentiment. The West Virginia Federation of Women's Clubs, along with the Daughters of the American Revolution and the West Virginia Christian Temperance Union, were enthusiastic supporters of the association and its campaign to deter workers from developing a strong class identity by fostering Americanization.[94]

The women's clubs were especially committed to Americanization programs. By the 1920s, the West Virginia Federation of Women's Clubs had established a special Americanization Department, and it prodded its local affiliates to sponsor regular Americanization programs. Concerned that the "melting pot [was] not melting," the state chairperson recommended that language and citizenship skills be promoted in every program the voluntary association held for the wives of working-class immigrants.[95]

Rising conservatism and a gradual rejection of reform ideals shaped the content of the programs women's clubs conducted in the 1920s. As affiliates of the American Constitutional Association, West Virginia clubs frequently hosted "four minute speakers" who modeled their presentations on the "Four Minute Men" who propagandized during World War I. These charismatic presenters offered pithy commentary on current political and social questions, always coming back to the need for loyalty to government and business.[96]

Class divisions and labor tensions discouraged women's reform efforts, but so did the popular culture of the day. As the concept of companionate marriage gained popularity, women were encouraged by magazines and popular experts to be intelligent and interesting to their husbands. Suddenly association with an auxiliary that supported one's husband's work was more attractive than enrollment in a women's club that sought to improve conditions for women and children. "Female fellowship," Sheila Rothman has written, "was a victim of romantic love."[97]

As clubwomen distanced themselves from reform efforts, Appalachian physicians, following national trends, began to alter their relationships with autonomous women's organizations and focus more of their support and attention on the activities of dependent women's auxiliaries. These agencies, begun in the early 1920s, gradually became the principal vehicles through which nonprofessional women promoted medical reform.

The Women's Auxiliary of the AMA, the parent organization of the Appalachian medical society auxiliaries, was established in 1922. Even before the national alliance was formed, a number of states had already witnessed the creation of women's subsidiaries to county and state medical societies. Members of these organizations sought to promote goodwill among physicians and encourage membership in local chapters of the AMA. The women who joined medical auxiliaries also recognized the important role they played in promoting the careers of their male family members by encouraging public obedience to the medical model.[98]

The women who organized at the AMA convention in St. Louis in 1922 did not present themselves as independent agents who wished to establish a new institution modeled on their own ideals. Instead, they graciously requested approval from the medical society's delegates before they proceeded with their enterprise.[99] The AMA's membership, after ensuring that it was assuming no financial responsibilities, quickly approved the women's request and permitted them to form the auxiliary.[100]

Most state medical associations had organized auxiliaries by 1930, and Appalachian states, like their counterparts, quickly witnessed the creation of gender-based subsidiaries. The female family members of physicians in Virginia organized in 1922, their counterparts in Kentucky followed the next year, and women in West Virginia joined them in 1925.[101] The first president of the West Virginia auxiliary was Minnie Laura Harris Rutherford, the wife of Dr. A. G. Rutherford, a native of Logan County who had worked as a company physician for years before moving to Huntington.[102]

It was clear from the very beginning that the existence of these women's auxiliaries depended on the goodwill, and even the permission, of their parent organizations. Kentucky's state auxiliary expressed its appreciation to the medical association for its "courtesy in allowing your wives, mothers and daughters to organize the Auxiliary."[103] The women of the Virginia subsidiary thanked their male partners for the "wonderful privilege you have granted us" and assured them that "we desire nothing more than to be asked to do something for the medical profession."[104] They constantly reminded physicians that their organization would pursue only the goals the physicians established for them and would not take any actions "contrary to, or independent of the Medical Society of Virginia."[105]

To determine what was in the best interests of the medical profession, auxiliary members sought guidance from members of their medical associations. The West Virginia auxiliary requested the establishment of an advisory board composed of three physicians in 1927. These doctors, the women insisted, were to be appointed by the president of the medical association.[106] Doctors who sat on this committee were expected to take an active role in guiding their cadet society. When the West Virginia State Women's Council, a benign coalition of female benevolent organizations, invited the medical society's subsidiary to join, the auxiliary members declined to accept until they could acquire permission from their male advisers.[107]

The auxiliary justified its deference to the medical profession by proclaiming the superiority of the character as well as the professional knowledge of the medical practitioner. Doctors were elevated above other men, the Virginia auxiliary proclaimed, through "heritage, education and experience."[108] "I believe," announced one member, that "my husband's profession [is] almost the greatest work a man can do."[109] Female supporters held the medical profession in such high regard that they believed they shared in its legitimacy. Since, as one associate wrote, "wives naturally absorb knowledge from their husbands," it was only appropriate that auxiliary members carry physicians' goals into the community to further their ambitions.[110]

Physicians reveled in the opportunities offered by this new vehicle. Unlike independent clubwomen, professional nurses, and settlement workers, auxiliary members did not claim legitimacy on the grounds of maternalism or professional credentials and professed no authority over health care policy except as the companions of medical practitioners. Although some doctors exhibited reservations about the auxiliary program early in its history, they quickly came to value the movement and adopted it as a conduit for carrying their message to the public.

The Virginia auxiliary, the first to be established in an Appalachian state, recognized that it could play an important role as a promoter of the medical association. Doctors contributed a page of their journal, the *Virginia Medical Monthly*, to the Women's Auxiliary, a trend soon emulated in other states. The women used the space to proclaim their plans for bestowing the "True Story of Medicine" on the community.[111]

Kentucky doctors were also conscious of the pivotal role the auxiliary could play in promoting their philosophy of medical care. In the October 1930 edition of its journal, the Kentucky State Medical Society praised the auxiliary and contemplated what appeared to it to be the great enthusiasm of the press for the women volunteers. "It is as interpreters of professional thought," the article proclaimed, "that the Auxiliary will find its greatest opportunity."[112] The next month, the editor returned to this topic and congratulated the auxiliary for the radio broadcasts it delivered in cooperation with the medical association. The writer once again applauded the ability of the auxiliary members to deliver the medical community's message in a clear and comprehensible fashion.[113]

The president of the Women's Auxiliary of the West Virginia State Medical Association reported to her colleagues in 1932 that they could best support the medical profession "through personal contacts, club work, the Hygiea Magazine, etc., keeping always before the public that the authority on health conditions is the medical man."[114] This declaration reminded auxiliary members of their subordinate role while affirming their unique mission as intimate allies and promoters of medical science.

Along with their general responsibility for convincing the community of the medical establishment's professional authority, auxiliary members were charged with steering independent women's clubs toward causes and programs acceptable to medical practitioners. This mission was spelled out in the resolution chartering the national auxiliary, which stated that the organization intended to "extend the aims of the medical profession through the wives of doctors to the various women's organizations which look to the advancement of health and education."[115]

Doctors' wives could be influential in women's clubs, the auxiliary reckoned, because as intimates of physicians they were often asked to serve on health care committees of their local women's clubs. To take advantage of this situation, auxiliary members were encouraged to use such positions to guarantee that independent clubs did not stray too far from the boundaries established by the medical associations.[116]

As part of a national campaign to encourage their sisters to evaluate the work of independent clubs, the members of the Women's Auxiliary of the AMA prepared an "Official Health Program" in 1930. This document critiqued the public health work of independent women's clubs and insisted that auxiliary members, as family relations of physicians, were the only females with the proper experience to guide such programs. It criticized clubwomen's projects as "fragmentary and ineffective" and asserted that "most volunteer agencies do not yet realize the wastefulness of their individualistic efforts."[117]

Medical associations maintained that this situation could be remedied if independent women's clubs would follow the guidance of medical auxiliary members. Through the involvement of auxiliary associates in women's clubs, doctors could be certain that independent volunteers fostered the ideals of the medical societies. Auxiliary members, for example, taught clubwomen that physicians were the final arbiters of public health and that volunteers and other citizens "should be willing to take orders from them."[118]

Instead of engaging in independent public health programs that challenged doctors' authority, auxiliary members promoted projects that increased the reliance of average citizens on physicians. They worked to achieve this goal in a number of ways, some of which were overt whereas others were subtle.

Radio broadcasts, a tactic used by all of the auxiliaries in the Appalachian region, proved to be a successful medium through which to promulgate this message. Women volunteers sponsored speakers such as the president of the Kentucky State Medical Society, who discussed his society's "contribution to Kentucky" in 1930.[119] At the May Day celebration in Letcher County, Kentucky, the Women's Auxiliary helped organize a parade that was marshaled by leaders of the state medical association and the state board of health. Bedecked with ribbons and flowers, the grandstand seemed more appropriate for a political campaign than a health lecture.[120]

In addition to promoting contemporary medical figures, the women's auxiliaries also venerated medical heroes. One of the primary projects of the Women's Auxiliary of the Kentucky State Medical Society was the Jane Todd Crawford Fund, a campaign to build a memorial to a mountain woman who had endured an ovariotomy without the benefit of anesthesia. The monument symbolized the triumph of modern scientific medicine and celebrated the skill of the surgeon, Ephraim McDowell, as well as the bravery of the patient.[121] Auxiliary members in eastern Kentucky were particularly enthusiastic about this project and announced that they had received great support from other women's organizations in their communities. Perry County, for example, reported that every women's group in Hazard had contributed to the fund-raising effort.[122]

Besides memorializing physicians, both living and dead, auxiliary members engaged in activities such as preparing flower arrangements for hospitals, sewing layettes for indigent families, and providing entertainment for convalescent children.[123] They did not, however, promote independent public health efforts, campaign to improve health care delivery for the indigent, or employ public health nurses. They clearly relinquished questions about health care delivery to their male associates.

In general, auxiliary members did their best to avoid matters that touched on the economics of health care. Their standard defense was that they were subordinate to the medical associations and that such issues were beyond their comprehension. When auxiliary members did take a stand on questions of medical economics, they were solidly in favor of their husbands' and fathers' positions.

On the question of private efforts to fund clinics for the needy, for example, the auxiliaries agreed with their male counterparts. "Free clinics conducted by unauthorized individuals are a menace to the profession," reported the *Kentucky Medical Journal*.[124] The Women's Auxiliary of the West Virginia State Medical Association responded enthusiastically when Dr. David Littlejohn of the West Virginia Public Health Association and later state health commissioner proclaimed that "we, instead of the laity, must take charge of Public Health."[125]

Auxiliary members shared the medical profession's opposition to large-scale federal funding of public health projects. In 1928, the women's auxiliaries, guided by the AMA, opposed a federal proposal aimed at securing supplemental funding for programs endangered by the withdrawal of Sheppard-Towner assistance. They requested that the federal government leave child welfare to the states, where physicians would be better able to administer and control the programs.[126] When a similar program was debated in 1929, auxiliaries were warned not to allow their associations to become centers for the distribution of propaganda. They were also instructed to discourage other women's organizations from supporting efforts of this sort.[127]

Physicians helped develop these dependent auxiliaries into the perfect propaganda machines. Embracing the ideal of companionate marriage and not maternalism, auxiliary members lacked an independent platform from which they could articulate a medical agenda separate from that of their professional family members. Unlike independent female activists who formed relationships with nurses and other public health promoters, the women's subsidiaries of county and state medical associations were formally bound to physicians. The fidelity they exhibited comforted doctors, who had watched their self-governing female supporters become too independent.

Physicians were willing to sacrifice the support they had previously received from autonomous women's groups because by the late 1920s they had begun to cement their long-standing bonds with state and local governments. During their crusades to eliminate sectarian practice and promote scientific medicine, physicians had grown increasingly dependent on the state to protect their professional privilege. The state, for its part, enthusiastically embraced the advances of modern medicine and wholeheartedly supported the physicians' efforts to establish a professional as well as an economic monopoly. The physicians' ability to reconcile the state's desire for a healthy citizenry with their own professional ambitions reduced the doctors' need to rely on nonprofessional advocates. With the punitive power of the government increasingly behind their efforts, physicians found themselves less dependent on the social transformation women activists assisted in creating.

Doctors also succeeded in limiting governmental and private support for autonomous public health programs. The termination of Sheppard-Towner funding in 1929, coupled with the turmoil of the Great Depression, shook the structures that had promoted progressive public health work in Appalachia. Threatened by the economic hardship of the depression, physicians labored to strengthen their own economic positions while gradually replacing nurses as the primary recipients of government funding for medical service. At the same time, private organizations that sustained innovative public health programs saw their unique reform initiatives supplanted by government programs that assumed a greater responsibility for the nation's social welfare. By the early 1930s, dependent auxiliaries of state and local medical societies were increasingly replacing independent women's organizations. Public health programs that had been initiated under the aegis of women's clubs or settlement schools became merely components of a formalized public health structure that limited the diversity of legitimate public health activities and promoted the proprietary medical model.[128]

CONCLUSION

Occupying the "free space" that Kathryn Kish Sklar, Seth Koven and Sonya Michel, Theda Skocpol, and Sara Evans and Harry Boyte have described between the state and the individual, clubwomen and settlement workers acted as the soft-spoken conscience of capitalism during industrialization in Appalachia.[1] They welcomed the economic and social opportunities made available to them as members of the middle or upper class but demanded at least minimal consideration of the conditions of mothers and children. At the same time, their activism was clearly defined by their own class position and their conviction that they, as middle-class Anglo-Saxon mothers, possessed the right as well as the obligation to improve the conditions under which working-class Appalachian women and their offspring lived and developed.[2]

Motivated by these objectives, women reformers moved to occupy an additional middle ground, this time between medical professionals and the populations they had yet to attract to their services. Female activists were resolute enthusiasts of scientific medical knowledge and committed maternalists determined to share the advantages of professional medical care with the women and children they had targeted for aid. As long as Appalachian physicians were struggling to define and fortify their own profession, the ambitions of the two constituencies coincided. When, however, the medical profession came to see these autonomous women's groups as threats to their sovereignty, they became resistant to what they perceived as a challenge. At the same time, women's groups were growing less interested in working-class mothers. In response to the labor unrest of the 1920s and the reactionary climate of the decade, women's voluntary associations gradually abandoned the middle ground between the state and working-class women and between physicians and impoverished women and children. Like many other American women, they turned inward to their own families and personal interests. Settlement workers, who continued to administer programs in rural counties, were increasingly defined by their developing professional identity, an identity that stressed objectivity over sentiment and denigrated the maternalism that had guided earlier work.[3]

When middle-class female reformers stopped advocating for the extension of medical programs to poor and working-class women and children, Sheila Rothman has argued, they gave up two tremendously important opportunities, a choice that had long-term consequences for all women and all Americans. By withdrawing from the public debate about medical care, they ensured that physicians confirmed their autonomy as the sole authorities qualified to speak about medicine. The demise of a popular conversation about medical services allowed doctors to usurp formerly public preventive care programs and secure them under the umbrella of proprietary medicine. Whereas Rothman sees these reverses in the context of the congressional defeat of the Sheppard-Towner Act, I argue that public discourse about medical programs ended at all levels and that the abandonment of health care advocacy by local and regional women reformers contributed mightily to the failure of the maternalist welfare state.[4]

Skocpol has written that the decline of maternalist identification and political activism in the 1920s prevented the creation of "a generous and caring American welfare state inherent in the maternalist policy breakthroughs of the Progressive Era and the early 1920s." With the collapse of middle-class, grassroots women's alliances in the 1920s, the possibility of tempering the professional ambition and autonomy of medical practitioners vanished. As class associates, women reformers were among the few people who could realistically serve as potential restraints on the growing power of medical professionals in the 1920s.[5] When women advocates withdrew from the public dialogue over the delivery of medical care, physicians successfully stymied the ability of nonprofessionals to speak as experts on health. Their professional prestige secure, doctors faced little opposition as they extended their public influence by co-opting government reform during the New Deal and into the World War II era.[6]

The potency of the physicians' strength and the absolute dominion they possessed over the delivery of medical care in Appalachia enabled the medical community to hold its own against the growing power of organized labor in the post–World War II era. Leading one of the strongest social forces in the region after World War II, the bosses of the United Mine Workers of America (UMWA) achieved a significant victory when they convinced the federal government to pressure coal operators into signing a contract establishing the union's Welfare and Retirement Fund in 1946.[7] Prompted by publication of a federal report that documented the desperate medical needs of Appalachian coal miners, the fund provided critically needed health services to residents of many isolated mining villages and helped displace the controversial company doctor system.[8] The program faced significant opposition from state medical societies and their parent, the American Medical Association, which finally terminated its recognition of the fund in 1958.[9]

The Kentucky State Medical Society and its allies in the state assembly demonstrated their impassioned antipathy toward the fund in a legislative fight that same year. Appalachian practitioners had long tolerated the intercession of the company between employees and contract doctors, but they viewed the fund as a direct challenge to their professional and social authority because it placed the power over medical finances in the hands of the union and not the company. In an effort to frustrate the fund's operations, state legislators, allied with the medical society, attempted to pass a law prohibiting out-of-state insurance companies from operating in Kentucky. The law, which was defeated, was a "bid by the state medical association to preserve the professional *status quo*" by denying recognition to a worker-controlled insurance company that challenged the hegemony of doctors and industrialists over workers.[10]

The Kentucky State Medical Society also objected to the fund's establishment of a series of hospitals across south-central Appalachia. The UMWA fund created the Miners' Memorial Hospital Association in 1951 and opened its first in-patient facility in 1956. Members of the state medical society contested the construction of these facilities and argued that union-affiliated hospitals competed unfairly with proprietary institutions owned by private physicians. They insisted that these new hospitals were redundant and would only serve to drive private practitioners out of business. Doctors voiced these protests in spite of the fact that the American Medical Association had documented the region's desperate need for modern hospitals in a confidential report commissioned in 1952.[11]

Throughout eastern Kentucky, county medical societies denied affiliation to doctors employed at UMWA facilities and demanded that medical society members disavow all professional association with those employed at the miners' hospitals. These actions, coupled with the changing economic conditions of the coal industry as large companies consolidated and mechanized, weakened the financial security of the hospitals, which were sold to the Board of National Missions of the Presbyterian Church, U.S.A., in 1963.[12]

Doctors were equally resistant to projects such as the Floyd County, Kentucky, Comprehensive Health Services Program launched in the 1960s. Initiated through the federal Office of Economic Opportunity, the program established community health centers intended to provide isolated or low-income citizens with access to medical care. These centers delivered the same sort of free or low-cost care that public health projects had provided during the first decades of the twentieth century. Just as those earlier programs had been labeled "state medicine" or "socialized medicine," doctors in Floyd County used similar appellations to condemn new initiatives created during the War on Poverty.[13]

By the 1960s and 1970s, however, increasing numbers of Appalachian citizens began to express their discontent with the medical system that professed to serve the region. Fueled by the civil rights movement and the campaign against black lung disease, Appalachian people began to reassess the quality of medical care available to them and question the philosophical arguments that legitimized the dominance of a health care system that failed to fully meet their needs.[14]

In part, changing economic conditions in the coalfields prompted this reevaluation. By the 1960s, physicians were significantly less interested in serving in the mountains of Appalachia than they had been a generation earlier. The region had endured a dramatic outmigration as a consequence of mechanization during the 1950s. At the same time, the UMWA Welfare and Retirement Fund had been depleted. As the population declined and the region's economic base deteriorated, few physicians chose to practice in rural areas.[15]

Unable to attract private physicians in the 1970s, small communities set out to secure federal monies and use the resources of the UMWA to extend the community health center effort initiated during the War on Poverty. The availability of private funds, whether guaranteed through deduction from workers' paychecks or sought through entrepreneurial activity, had initially attracted physicians to the mountains. By the 1970s, however, mountain residents possessed few monetary resources and relied instead on government assistance and private grant monies. As brokers of outside funds, activists who administered programs like the Mud Creek Clinic, the Clover Fork Clinic, and the Big Sandy Area Health Care Cor-

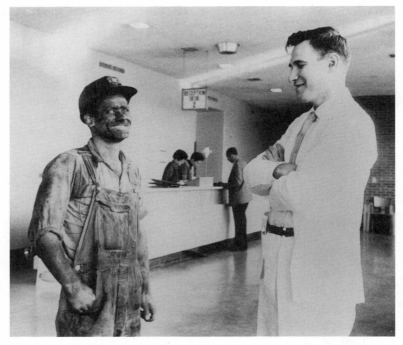

As indicated by the striking difference in appearance between this coal miner and this physician, a medical system that elevated doctors above patients was well established by World War II. West Virginia and Regional History Collection, West Virginia University.

poration managed to bring critical primary care services to many country folk.[16]

Ironically, many of the leaders who helped spark the creation of these clinics and demanded recognition of black lung disease were working-class women. Eula Hall, for example, was an impoverished mother who grew "tired of being pushed around" and led a campaign to support the Mud Creek Clinic.[17] Descended from the women targeted by middle-class reformers in the 1920s, these wives and daughters of coal miners and other workers imbibed the democratic rhetoric of the 1960s and demanded reform of the medical system in rural Appalachia.[18]

These projects were shaped by democratic ideals and the stated intention of including local residents in both the planning and the implementation of all major decisions. Such efforts were often undermined by a class structure that devalued poor rural people and the continued belief that medical practitioners enjoyed special rights that placed their interests above those of the population seeking service. In spite of projects such as the National Health Service Corps, a program based on the belief that all Americans, with the aid of government, should have access to a physician, "public programs are [still] premised on control by physicians."[19]

Just as industrialization transformed Appalachian residents into valued workers worthy of medical care, the processes of deindustrialization determined that they had ceased to possess significant market value. As a surplus labor force, Appalachian people could no longer rely on private capital to support their health care infrastructure. Without the financial guarantees provided by private capital, the proprietary medical profession, in general, was no longer willing to provide health care to mountain people.[20]

When physicians terminated their practices and were not replaced by new practitioners, the people of Appalachia found themselves in an ironic but tragic position. Doctors who had once flooded the region, warning the government and private citizens alike that they alone were qualified to provide medical services, were no longer willing to dispense the skills over which they had acquired a monopoly. The region's inhabitants, therefore, were forced to entreat physicians to deliver services that doctors and middle-class reformers had convinced them they needed less than a century earlier.[21]

In response to this situation, some Appalachian people have attempted to revive preindustrial traditions to provide caregivers to communities no longer served by physicians. The battle to repeal the laws prohibiting lay midwifery in West Virginia in the early 1990s reminds us that the transformation of Appalachian medicine eighty years ago still has significant consequences today.

In 1992, fifty obstetricians served a population of slightly under 2 million people in West Virginia. Including nurse-midwives and other physicians who delivered babies, approximately 100 practitioners were qualified to assist mothers in childbirth. The vast majority of these practitioners were located in Morgantown, Wheeling, Charleston, Huntington, and Beckley. Many of the state's fifty-five counties had no obstetrical providers at all.[22]

In 1972, the state had rewritten its midwifery laws to discourage home births by prohibiting midwives from accepting fees for assisting in deliveries. Although the law was in effect for twenty years before a move was initiated to change it, legislative restriction did not end the practice of lay midwifery and the occurrence of home births. In the 1970s and 1980s, young families who lived in many of the state's rural counties continued to deliver their children at home with the assistance of midwives. Many of these families had recently arrived in Appalachia as part of a back-to-the-land movement begun during the 1960s.

In the early 1980s, a group of about a dozen lay midwives practicing in West Virginia established the Midwives Alliance of West Virginia, a state affiliate of the Midwives Alliance of North America. Through this organization, they sought to police their practices and pursue ongoing educational opportunities for themselves and other potential midwives. Some of the midwives enjoyed cordial relations with physicians who supported their practices; others lacked such support.[23]

The members of the Midwives Alliance determined that they should seek regulation from the state in the early 1990s. Many specters from the Progressive Era appeared in the 1992 battle over licensing lay midwives. Just as the state medical associations had led the fight against lay midwives in the Progressive Era, so too did the West Virginia State Medical Association head the crusade against licensing lay midwives in the 1990s. The president of the association rejected proposals for physician supervision of midwives and insisted that "an obstetrician is the gold standard of care. I don't think anyone would argue the best quality of care would come from an obstetrician."[24]

As the physicians condemned the midwives, observers recognized the self-interest inherent in their message. The editor of the *Charleston Gazette*, the newspaper of record for the state, warned that the medical association was resisting because "doctors want to retain their monopoly on the medical gold mine."[25] The female senator who sponsored the bill complained that "some of the doctors who have been down here lobbying against [the bill] don't even take poor patients. They're the ones who are motivated by greed."[26]

If the confrontation between midwives and doctors recalls tensions first enunciated seventy-five years earlier, the attitudes of the women who opposed the bill in the assembly illustrate the absolute conviction with which many middle-class and elite women have internalized their dependence on educated medical professionals.

A Republican delegate who was married to a physician expressed concerns about lay midwives' level of education. When she argued that she did not "believe in watch one, do one, and teach one," she dismissed the traditional knowledge acquired by empirical practitioners through the centuries and deferred to the standard of formal medical education that developed at the end of the nineteenth century.[27]

The issue was less about education than it was about economics for a delegate from Charleston. Barter between two rural women did not concern the female official, but the possibility that midwives might bill the state's employees' insurance fund did. "We're talking about economics. We're talking about licensing women who are not educated. We're talking about billing PEIA [the state employees' insurance plan]. We're talking about risk!"[28]

The actions of the delegate married to the physician affirm the hegemony of the medical presumptions articulated in the 1920s and their resonance through the decades. As the wife of a doctor, she had fully incorporated the convictions first announced during the Progressive Era. For her, protecting women and infants meant saving them from uneducated healers.

During the legislative debate, she distributed a letter from her husband's medical practice that described the difficulty faced by a young mother who had been preparing for childbirth with an Ohio midwife. According to newspaper reports, the letter indicated that because of her reliance on a midwife, the mother was about to give birth to a handicapped child. The newspaper writer who was covering the midwifery debate published a story stating that the letter failed to mention that the child had been born healthy a few days before the bill came to the floor for a final vote.[29]

The motives of the delegate who introduced the letter were not revealed in the newspaper account, but her deeds stand as a dramatic symbol of the accomplishment of the medical profession in co-opting women activists to their cause. Although an elected official able to speak in her own right, she used her husband's experience as a medical practitioner as ammunition in her battle to defeat this bill. Holding up a medical specialist as "the gold standard" of care, she was convinced that any tactic was valid in her effort to protect women and babies from incompetent midwives. If her actions helped safeguard her husband's profession, so much the better.

The defeat of the midwifery bill in West Virginia illustrates the perpetuation of tensions since the Progressive Era, but it also demonstrates how successful physicians have been in convincing the public, especially women, that no other legitimate practitioners should be allowed to compete with them. As a small group of nonprofessionals who lacked strong grassroots support, West Virginia's lay midwives had little in common with the middle- and upper-class women who might have supported them in the legislature. The inability of these women to ally or even communicate across class and professional lines suggests that Theda Skocpol is correct when she argues that "contemporary feminists may also be able to learn lessons from the maternalists of old who, in their self conceptions and public rhetoric, stressed solidarity between privileged and less privileged women, and honor for values of caring and nurturance," values that have been denigrated by the medical model that emerged seventy-five years ago.[30]

NOTES

Abbreviations

The following abbreviations are used in the notes.

CFC — Claude Frazier Collection, Eastern Regional Coal Archives, Craft Memorial Library, Bluefield, W.Va.

ERCA — Eastern Regional Coal Archives, Craft Memorial Library, Bluefield, W.Va.

GFWCWHRC — General Federation of Women's Clubs Women's History and Resource Center, Washington, D.C.

KHSL — Kornhauser Health Sciences Library, University of Louisville, Louisville, Ky.

KMJ — *Kentucky Medical Journal*

KSDLA — Kentucky State Department of Libraries and Archives, Frankfort, Ky.

LNC — Linda Neville Collection, Special Collections, M. I. King Library, University of Kentucky, Lexington, Ky.

MCVA — Medical College of Virginia Archives, Tompkins-McCaw Library, Richmond, Va.

MIKL — Special Collections, M. I. King Library, University of Kentucky, Lexington, Ky.

NARA — National Archives and Records Administration, Washington, D.C.

SAA — Southern Appalachian Archives, Hutchins Library, Berea College, Berea, Ky.

SHC — Sanger Historical Collection, RG 61, Medical College of Virginia Archives, Tompkins-McCaw Library, Richmond, Va.

USPHSC — U.S. Public Health Service Collection, RG 90, National Archives and Records Administration, Washington, D.C.

VMM — *Virginia Medical Monthly*

VSA — Virginia State Archives, Richmond, Va.

WPAHMKC — Works Progress Administration History of Medicine in Kentucky Collection, Kornhauser Health Sciences Library, University of Louisville, Louisville, Ky.

WVMJ — *West Virginia Medical Journal*

WVRHC — West Virginia and Regional History Collection, West Virginia University, Morgantown, W.Va.

WVSMAH — West Virginia State Medical Association Headquarters, Charleston, W.Va.

Introduction

1. West Virginia Federation of Women's Clubs, *Yearbook*, 1931–32, 33.

2. "Advantages of Organized Efforts among the Women," *VMM* 53, no. 4 (July 1926): 265.

3. Leavitt, *Healthiest City*, 190–213. Leavitt discusses the importance of voluntary organization in promoting health reform in an urban environment during the same era.

4. Borst, *Catching Babies*. Borst's examination of the displacement of midwives by general practitioners in Wisconsin follows very similar developments during roughly the same time period.

5. Anglin, "Lives on the Margin"; Jane Becker, *Selling Tradition*; Maggard, "Class and Gender," "From the Farm to the Coal Camp," and "Gender, Race, and Place"; Smith, *Women of the Rural South*, and *Digging Our Own Graves*; Tice, "School-Work and Mother-Work."

6. Ladd-Taylor, *Mother-Work*; Koven and Michel, *Mothers of a New World* and "Womanly Duties"; Skocpol, *Protecting Soldiers and Mothers*.

7. Skocpol, *Protecting Soldiers and Mothers*, 36.

8. Smith, "Walk-ons in the Third Act," 6.

9. On the position of Appalachia in the nineteenth-century economy, see Dunaway, *First American Frontier*; Lewis, *Transforming the Appalachian Countryside*; Inscoe, *Mountain Masters*; Pudup, "Limits of Subsistence"; and Herrin, "Breaking the Stillness." For comparative studies of the development of commercial production, see, for example, Hahn, *Roots of Southern Populism*; Hahn and Prude, *Countryside in the Age of Capitalist Transformation*; Kulikoff, "Transformation to Capitalism"; Prude, *Coming of the Industrial Order*; and Rothenberg, "Emergence of Farm Labor Markets."

10. Lewis, "Appalachian Restructuring"; Gaventa, *Power and Powerlessness*; Ronald Eller, *Miners, Millhands, and Mountaineers*. See Waller's *Feud* for an exhaustive study of change in one limited geographical area.

11. Dunaway, *First American Frontier*; Noe, *Southwest Virginia's Railroads*; Salstrom, "Newer Appalachia"; Inscoe, *Mountain Masters*; Lewis, *Transforming the Appalachian Countryside*, 51–52, 256.

12. Pudup, "Boundaries of Class"; Pudup, Billings, and Waller, *Appalachia in the Making*.

13. Billings, Pudup, and Waller, "Taking Exception with Exceptionalism," 17–18.

14. Warner, "Ideals of Science," 464.

15. Matriculation Book, 1838–71, MCVA.

16. Ely, *The Big Sandy*, 154–55, 182–87, 300–302, 437, 444–45; Fuson, *History of Bell County*, 538–59. For a comparison with nineteenth-century physicians from outside the region, see Leavitt, " 'Worrying Profession.' "

17. Ely, *The Big Sandy*, 154, 186; Callahan, *History of West Virginia*, 2:155, 521; 3:431.

18. Letters—Miscellaneous, 1859–89, SHC; "The Early Physicians of the Sandy River District," #92159, CFC.

19. Dunaway, *First American Frontier*, 320–22; Starr, *Social Transformation of American Medicine*, 65–67. Dunaway has offered overwhelming evidence to illustrate that Appalachia was already connected to outside markets before the industrial era. Her argument that such ties only served to impoverish most Appalachian residents supports my claim that professional medicine had little impact in rural Appalachia before the Civil War since, as Starr has discussed, the services of a doctor were rarely secured by poor, rural people, who tended to rely on resources within the household for medical care.

20. Starr, *Social Transformation of American Medicine*, 76.

21. Ronald Eller, *Miners, Millhands, and Mountaineers*; Corbin, *Life, Work, and Rebellion*; Trotter, *Coal, Class, and Color*.

22. Weiner, "Middlemen of the Coalfields," 32. Physicians who moved to Appalachia to take advantage of the region's economic expansion reflect some of the characteristics of the young Jewish immigrants Weiner has described who came to Appalachia during the same era. Like these Jewish merchants, physicians were both pushed to move to the region by excessive competition in more commercially oriented areas and pulled by the growth of the region's economy. Just as the Jewish merchants possessed special knowledge of the garment industry that enabled them to secure positions in developing town economies, so, too, did physicians seek economic status and social acceptance based on their unique knowledge.

23. Warner, *Therapeutic Perspective*, 31, 80, 254–57.

24. Borst, *Catching Babies*, 91.

25. Ludmerer, *Learning to Heal*, 35, 49–51; Warner, *Therapeutic Perspective*, 243; Bonner, *Becoming a Physician*, 276–77.

26. Ellis, *Medicine in Kentucky*, 15.

27. Flexner, *Medical Education in the United States and Canada*, 229–31, 238–39, 315–16; Norwood, *Medical Education in the United States before the Civil War*, 223–41, 269–75, 298–303; Ludmerer, *Learning to Heal*, 98; "1907–08 Merger Brought U of L Diploma Problems," Curriculum Reform File, Catalogs and Announcements, KHSL. Although it has been successfully argued that the reform of medical education began well before the publication of the Flexner report, it is still noteworthy that Flexner roundly criticized all three of these institutions in his review of medical education throughout the United States and Canada.

28. Pudup, "Town and Country," 286.

29. Starr, *Social Transformation of American Medicine*, 60.

30. Contemporary biographical sources provide many examples of local physicians who succeeded in acquiring positions with railroads or mines or who invested in such enterprises. See Callahan, *History of West Virginia*, 2:134, 138, 157, 234–35, 238, 241, 370, 378, 471, 497–98, 521, 545, 576, 596; 3:22, 56, 139, 211, 603. On the importance of acquiring formal education outside the mountains as an economic strategy, see Maggard, "From Farmers to Miners," 39.

31. Rothstein, *American Physicians*, 288.

32. Friedson, *Professional Dominance*, 147.

33. Larson, *Rise of Professionalism*. James Scott offers a critically important view of class identification in *Domination and the Arts of Resistance*, 67.

34. Friedson, "Are the Professions Necessary?," 15.

35. Bledstein, *Culture of Professionalism*, 4.

36. Friedson, "Are the Professions Necessary?," 10–21.

37. Rosenberg, *No Other Gods*, 12–13.

38. Blee and Billings, "Family Strategies," 69; Shifflet, *Coal Towns*, 23; Pudup, "Town and Country," 286.

39. Starr, *Social Transformation of American Medicine*, 66.

40. Kentucky State Register of Physicians, 1847, 1852, WPAHMKC; Pudup, "Land before Coal," 263–74; Pudup, "Town and Country," 287. Surveys conducted by the commonwealth of Kentucky during the 1840s and 1850s revealed that no doctors lived in several eastern Kentucky counties. Research by geographer Mary Beth Pudup has documented the absence or scarcity of physicians in eastern Kentucky from the middle of the century through 1880.

41. McMillen, *Motherhood in the Old South*, 8–9; Hoffert, *Private Matters*, 62; Borst, *Catching Babies*, 5.

42. Leavitt, *Typhoid Mary*, 35.

43. Higginbotham, "From Our Mountain Nurses," 28.

44. Starr, *Social Transformation of American Medicine*, 94–100.

45. Leavitt, *Healthiest City*, 80, 112; *Typhoid Mary*, 34–35, 46–47; and "'Typhoid Mary' Strikes Back," 629; "Once More into the Breach," *Jackson Hustler*, 10 January 1902; "Biennial Bulletins of the State Board of Health of Kentucky" and "Kentucky Medical History, 1801–1940," WPAHMKC. Leavitt's studies of public health in Milwaukee and of Typhoid Mary demonstrate that such dialogues were not unique to Appalachia. Numerous examples of the debates over the treatment of smallpox and over the effectiveness of vaccination can be found in the reports sent by county health officers to the State Board of Health of Kentucky, WPAHMKC.

46. Bledstein, *Culture of Professionalism*, 35.

47. Larson, "Production of Expertise," 34.

48. Borst, *Catching Babies*; Donegan, *Women and Men Midwives*; Leavitt, *Brought to Bed*; Litoff, *American Midwives*; Wertz and Wertz, *Lying-in*.

49. Brickman, "Public Health, Midwives, and Nurses," 74.

50. Borst, *Catching Babies*, 126–30. Unlike the physicians who used shared immigrant status to ease their way into the birthing rooms of Wisconsin mothers, Appalachian physicians seldom shared ethnic identities with their patients.

51. Skocpol, *Protecting Soldiers and Mothers*, 321–39. On the development of women's organizations and their importance in American political and social life, see Baker, "Domestication of Politics"; Anne Firor Scott, *Natural Allies*; Blair, *Clubwoman as Feminist*; and Bordin, *Women and Temperance*.

52. Sklar, "Historical Foundations of Women's Power," 69.

53. Ladd-Taylor and Umansky, *"Bad" Mothers*, 9; Koven and Michel, "Womanly Duties," 1078; Tice, "School-Work and Mother-Work," 196.

54. Skocpol, *Protecting Soldiers and Mothers*, 482, 683, n. 9; Muncy, *Creating a*

Female Dominion. Like Skocpol, I believe that the work of local and regional women's groups was critical to the functioning of the female reform elite described by Muncy.

55. Pudup, "Town and Country," 292.

56. Meckel, *Save the Babies*, 152.

57. Cott, *Grounding of Modern Feminism*, 193–96; Anne Firor Scott, *Natural Allies*, 180. Cott has described the debates that developed around marriage and career in the 1920s. I would suggest that a career as a volunteer, in this context, provided middle-class women with a way to elevate their family condition, both economically and socially, while avoiding the tensions that could arise if women actually accepted paid employment outside the home.

58. McMillen, *Motherhood in the Old South*, 183; Lebsock, *Free Women of Petersburg*, 169–70. As both McMillen and Lebsock have pointed out, middle- and upper-class women were the most likely candidates to embrace physicians as childbirth attendants in the American South.

59. Hewitt, *Women's Activism and Social Change*, 44; Ginzberg, *Women and the Work of Benevolence*.

60. Sklar, "Historical Foundations of Women's Power," 45; Muncy, *Creating a Female Dominion*, 3–37.

61. Sklar, "Hull House in the 1890s," 658–59; Muncy, *Creating a Female Dominion*.

62. For general introductions to the settlement movement in America, see Carson, *Settlement Folk*; Chambers, *Seedtime of Reform*; Davis, *Spearheads for Reform*; Lubove, *Professionalism and Altruism*; and Trolander, *Professionalism and Social Change*. Specific studies of African American and immigrant settlement experiences can be found in Lasch-Quinn, *Black Neighbors*, and Lissak, *Pluralism and Progressives*. For information on settlement schools in Appalachia, see Whisnant, *All That Is Native and Fine*; Forderhase, "Eve Returns to the Garden"; and Tice, "School-Work and Mother-Work."

63. Whisnant, *All That Is Native and Fine*, 33–34; Tice, "School-Work and Mother-Work," 196.

64. Carson, *Settlement Folk*, 135–38; Whisnant, *All That Is Native and Fine*, 43.

65. Tice, "School-Work and Mother-Work," 194–97, 216.

66. Higginbotham, "From Our Mountain Nurses," 28; "Dream Houses," box 74, LNC.

67. Breckinridge, *Wide Neighborhoods*; Dye, "Mary Breckinridge."

68. "Midwifery" License, Mary Breckinridge, 1924, Registry of Physicians and Nurses, Leslie County Court Records, microfilm, KSDLA.

69. Melosh, "*Physician's Hand*"; Reverby, *Ordered to Care*; Buhler-Wilkerson, *False Dawn*. Muncy's outstanding description of the different attitudes men and women articulated about professionalization can be found in *Creating a Female Dominion*, 124–57.

70. Ladd-Taylor, *Mother-Work*, 177–80; Skocpol, *Protecting Soldiers and Mothers*, 510; Muncy, *Creating a Female Dominion*, 134–42.

71. Rothman, *Woman's Proper Place*, 142; Skocpol, *Protecting Soldiers and Mothers*, 515; Meckel, *Save the Babies*, 217.

72. Sklar, "Call for Comparisons," 1113.

73. Rothman, *Woman's Proper Place*, 177–218; Skocpol, *Protecting Soldiers and Mothers*, 517–19; Cott, *Grounding of Modern Feminism*, 143–74; Maggard, "From Farmers to Miners," 40.

74. Hennen, *Americanization of West Virginia*, 119–34.

Chapter One

1. Arnow, *Dollmaker*, 10–12.

2. Starr, *Social Transformation of American Medicine*, 68–69.

3. Cassedy, "Why Self-Help?"

4. Leavitt, " 'Worrying Profession,' " provides comparison with a Wisconsin physician from the same era.

5. Ely, *The Big Sandy*, 437.

6. Ronald Eller, *Miners, Millhands, and Mountaineers*, 128–60.

7. Warner, *Therapeutic Perspective*, 6–7.

8. Butler, *Medical Register*; Polk, *Medical and Surgical Directory*, 1886; Starr, *Social Transformation of American Medicine*, 140.

9. Shaunna Scott, *Two Sides to Everything*, 8–9.

10. Pudup, "Land before Coal," 263–74, and "Town and Country," 287.

11. Dunaway, *First American Frontier*, 21.

12. Ibid., 294.

13. Pudup, "Town and Country," 286, and "Land before Coal," 154.

14. Board of Health of the State of West Virginia, *Biennial Report*, 1887–88, 23–45; Rothstein, *American Medical Schools*, 48–49, 55–56.

15. Rothstein, *American Medical Schools*, 49; Bonner, *Becoming a Physician*, 176–79.

16. Matriculation Book, 1838–71, MCVA.

17. Bonner, *Becoming a Physician*, 175–79, 217–25.

18. Norwood, *Medical Education in the United States before the Civil War*, 271–72.

19. Membership Records, 1900–1925, WVSMAH; Deceased Files, Virginia State Board of Medicine, Richmond, Va.; Polk, *Medical and Surgical Directory*, 1886, *Medical and Surgical Register*, 1896, *Medical Register*, 1906, 1917.

20. *Louisville Directory* for 1848–1849, Catalogs and Announcements, KHSL; Rothstein, *American Medical Schools*, 95.

21. Flexner, *Medical Education in the United States and Canada*, 229, 235, 315. The Medical College of Virginia did receive a small annual stipend from the state, but the vast majority of its costs were covered by student fees.

22. Starr, *Social Transformation of American Medicine*, 44–45.

23. T. R. Fulton to Levin Joynes, 26 September 1886, Letters—Miscellaneous, 1859–89, SHC.

24. I. G. Haller to Levin Joynes, 20 September 1870, Letters—Miscellaneous, 1859–89, SHC.

25. Applications for Medical Licenses, 1890–1925, unprocessed collection, KSDLA.

26. Polk, *Medical and Surgical Directory*, 1886, *Medical and Surgical Register*, 1896, *Medical Register*, 1906, 391–406, 913–29, 940–45.

27. Board of Health of the State of West Virginia, *Biennial Report*, 1887–88, 23–45.

28. Ritchie, "Infant Mortality."

29. "The Early Physicians of the Sandy River District," #92159, CFC; Matriculation Book, 1838–71, MCVA.

30. Applications for Medical Licenses, 1890–1925, unprocessed collection, KSDLA.

31. A. J. Robards to Simon Buckner, 8 September 1889, quoted in Pearce, *Days of Darkness*, 4. Compare both the writing and the environment of Wisconsin's rural physicians with those of eastern Kentucky's physicians. See Leavitt, " 'Worrying Profession.' "

32. Applications for Medical Licenses, 1890–1925, unprocessed collection, KSDLA; Ely, *The Big Sandy*, 154, 183, 185–87.

33. I. M. Repass to Levin Joynes, 16 December 1869, Letters—Miscellaneous, 1859–89, SHC.

34. I. G. Haller to Levin Joynes, 20 September 1870, Letters—Miscellaneous, 1859–89, SHC.

35. William Terry to Levin Joynes, 30 June, 29 July 1870, Letters—Miscellaneous, 1859–89, SHC.

36. Rothstein, *American Medical Schools*, 67; Warner, *Therapeutic Perspective*, 80, 95–97.

37. See Warner, "Ideals of Science" and *Therapeutic Perspective*, 162–84.

38. Luther Buford, "Fever Which Prevailed in Lancaster, Kentucky, 1835–36," Fevers and Folk Medicine before 1900, file 17, box 13, WPAHMKC.

39. Ibid.; Warner, *Therapeutic Perspective*, 100–101.

40. Luther Buford, "Fever Which Prevailed in Lancaster, Kentucky, 1835–36," Fevers and Folk Medicine before 1900, file 17, box 13, WPAHMKC.

41. "The Medical Society Declare That the Mortality of Middlesboro Is Less Than in Most Any City Its Size," Bell County Medical Society Records, 1890–1922, file 32, box 8, WPAHMKC.

42. "The Early Physicians of the Sandy River District," #92159, CFC; Warner, *Therapeutic Perspective*, 144–45.

43. Warner, *Therapeutic Perspective*, 169. Warner argues that apprenticeship was the most conservative method of medical education. Since so many Appalachian physicians were trained in this fashion, it should be of little surprise that antiquated concepts were retained.

44. Miles, *Spirit of the Mountains*, 24.

45. Leonard Roberts, *Up Cutshin and Down Greasy*, 95; Shackelford and Weinberg, *Our Appalachia*, 127.

46. Lopes, Moser, and Perkinson, *Appalachian Folk Medicine*, 13–15.

47. Johnson, *Narrative History of Wise County*, 354.

48. Ely, *The Big Sandy*, 437; Crellin and Philpott, *Trying to Give Ease*, 16–17; Shelley and Evans, "Women Folk Healers," 212; Rosenberg, "Therapeutic Revolution," 9.

49. Lopes, Moser, and Perkinson, *Appalachian Folk Medicine*, 45.

50. Leonard Roberts, *Up Cutshin and Down Greasy*, 97; Lopes, Moser, and Perkinson, *Appalachian Folk Medicine*, 41–42, 44.

51. Miles, *Spirit of the Mountains*, 25.

52. Higginbotham, "From Our Mountain Nurses," 28.

53. Shelley and Evans, "Women Folk Healers," 212.

54. Furman, *Sight to the Blind*, 44–46.

55. Campbell, *Southern Highlander*, 208–10.

56. Mrs. Arthur T. McCormack, "Our Pioneer Heroine of Surgery—Mrs. Jane Todd Crawford," *VMM* 61, no. 4 (July 1934): 231–32. In 1809, when eastern Kentucky was still a frontier, Jane Todd Crawford's family sought the help of a professionally trained physician to induce the delivery of the infant she appeared to be carrying. Upon examination of the forty-six-year-old mother of four, Dr. Ephraim McDowell determined that she was not pregnant but instead suffered from a foreign growth in her abdomen. To relieve her condition, he proposed that she travel the sixty miles to his office in Danville to undergo a radically experimental surgery. Crawford submitted to the operation, and, without the use of anesthesia, McDowell removed a twenty-two-pound tumor from her body while she recited Bible verses and male family members restrained her.

57. Stage, *Female Complaints*, 27.

58. Leonard Roberts, *Up Cutshin and Down Greasy*, 96.

59. "State vs. Ragland," in Board of Health of the State of West Virginia, *Biennial Report*, 1887–88, 65–68.

60. Ronald Eller, *Miners, Millhands, and Mountaineers*, xxi.

61. Gaventa, *Power and Powerlessness*, 54.

62. Banks, "Class Formation," 338–40; Corbin, *Life, Work, and Rebellion*, 142–43.

63. Veazey, *First Annual Report*, 7–9, 74.

64. Herrin, "Breaking the Stillness," 3.

65. Hibbard, *Virginia Coal*, 10.

66. Shaunna Scott, *Two Sides to Everything*, 7–8.

67. Paul, *Nineteenth Annual Report*, 41; Laing, *Annual Report*, 83.

68. Jillson, *Coal Industry in Kentucky*, 158.

69. Hibbard, *Virginia Coal*, 89, 107, 116, 125, 140–41, 150–51.

70. U.S. Department of Commerce, Bureau of the Census, *Thirteenth Census of the United States Taken in the Year 1910*, vol. 3, *Population, 1910, Reports by States, with Statistics for Counties, Cities, and Other Civil Divisions*, 1018–24.

71. "Comparative Birth Rate Standings of Counties and Cities," in *Annual Report of the State Board of Health and the State Health Commission to the Governor of Virginia for the Fiscal Year Ending September 30, 1919*, 102; Corbin, *Life, Work, and Rebellion*, 62–63.

72. Laing, *Annual Report*, 306, 334–35.

73. Frazier and Brown, *Miners and Medicine*, 65.

74. Rakes, "West Virginia's Entrepreneurial Alliance."

75. Beardsley, *History of Neglect*, 12.

76. McGehee, "Sawbones," 11.

77. Mulcahy, "New Deal for the Coal Miners," 31.

78. Weiner, "Middlemen of the Coalfields," 40.

79. Banks, "Class Formation," 343.

80. Dunaway, First American Frontier, 262; Keith, Country People, 180–82.

81. Pudup, "Boundaries of Class"; Maggard, "From Farmers to Miners."

82. Callahan, History of West Virginia, 3:431.

83. Ibid., 2:521.

84. Ibid., 2:576.

85. Waller, Feud, 158–81, 243; Callahan, History of West Virginia, 3:23–24.

86. "The Early Physicians of the Sandy River District," #92159, CFC.

87. Applications for Medical Licenses, 1890–1925, unprocessed collection, KSDLA.

88. "The Early Physicians of the Sandy River District," #92159, CFC; Lewis, Transforming the Appalachian Countryside, 256–57.

89. "The Early Physicians of the Sandy River District," #92159, CFC.

90. Shifflet, Coal Towns, 23.

91. Corbin, Life, Work, and Rebellion, 135.

92. "The Early Physicians of the Sandy River District," #92159, CFC.

93. Rothstein, American Medical Schools, 92. Rothstein has found that the number of medical schools grew from 65 in 1860 to 100 in 1880 and 160 in 1900. The number of graduates increased accordingly.

94. Polk, Medical and Surgical Directory, 1886, Medical and Surgical Register, 1896, Medical Register, 1906. These are conservative estimates since they are based on replies from physicians practicing in 1906. They do not include physicians who practiced in the region but relocated before Polk's survey was conducted.

95. Polk, Medical and Surgical Directory, 1886, 391–404.

96. Bonner, Becoming a Physician, 294; Rothstein, American Medical Schools, 142–43.

97. Membership Records, 1900–1925, WVSMAH.

98. Polk, Medical and Surgical Register, 1896, 1527, 1529, 1534.

99. Callahan, History of West Virginia, 2:109, 242, 623.

100. "The Early Physicians of the Sandy River District," #92159, CFC.

101. Polk, Medical and Surgical Directory, 1886, Medical and Surgical Register, 1896, Medical Register, 1906, 1917.

102. Ibid.

103. Lewis, Transforming the Appalachian Countryside, 194, 199.

104. Kegley, Wythe County, 105.

105. Henry D. Hatfield to Walter S. Hallanan, 15 June 1929, A&M #1661, Henry D. Hatfield Collection, WVRHC.

106. Stuart McGehee, "A Century of Care: A History of Bluefield Regional Medical Center, Bluefield Community Hospital, Bluefield Sanitarium," unpublished manuscript, ERCA.

107. Ibid.

108. "Hospitalization Facilities of the Region," Bluefield Daily Telegraph, 14 December 1939.

109. Stuart McGehee, "A Century of Care: A History of Bluefield Regional

Medical Center, Bluefield Community Hospital, Bluefield Sanitarium," unpublished manuscript, ERCA.

110. Flexner, *Medical Education in the United States and Canada*, 237.

111. Callahan, *History of West Virginia*, 3:23–24.

Chapter Two

1. Friedson, "Are the Professions Necessary?," 10; Starr, *Social Transformation of American Medicine*, 134–35; Borst, *Catching Babies*, 91; Warner, *Therapeutic Perspective*, 31, 80, 254–57.

2. Rothstein, *American Medical Schools*; Ludmerer, *Learning to Heal*, 98.

3. Starr, *Social Transformation of American Medicine*, 90–91, 99; Warner, "Ideals of Science," 464.

4. Leavitt, *Healthiest City*, esp. chap. 3.

5. Rosenkrantz, "Cart before Horse," 58.

6. Ibid., 58, 61, 62; Keith, *Country People*. Keith describes the consequences of state intrusion through road construction and education in the Upper Cumberland of Tennessee during this same era.

7. Friedson, "Are the Professions Necessary?," 16.

8. Ludmerer, *Learning to Heal*, 46–56; Rothstein, *American Medical Schools*, 98–99, 103–9; Borst, *Catching Babies*, 94.

9. Membership Records, 1900–1925, WVSMAH.

10. Polk, *Medical and Surgical Register*, 1896, *Medical Register*, 1906, 1917.

11. Borst, "Wisconsin's Midwives," 90–116.

12. Norwood, *Medical Education in the United States before the Civil War*, 275.

13. Minutes, Meeting of the Faculty of the Medical College of Virginia, 27 November 1893, MCVA.

14. Flexner, *Medical Education in the United States and Canada*, 229 (emphasis in original).

15. Ibid.

16. Ibid., 236.

17. Ibid., 239; Rothstein, *American Medical Schools*, 146; Bonner, *Becoming a Physician*, 304.

18. "1907–08 Merger Brought U of L Diploma Problems," Curriculum Reform File, Catalogs and Announcements, KHSL. Initially, this merger created difficulties because less well prepared students from the proprietary schools had to compete with more highly qualified University of Louisville students.

19. University of Louisville Medical Department, *Fifty-ninth Annual Announcement, Session of 1895–96*, Catalogs and Announcements, KHSL; Mary Kay Becker, "Medical Education in Kentucky prior to 1910," unpublished paper in author's possession.

20. Minutes, Meeting of the Faculty of the Medical College of Virginia, 27 November 1893, MCVA.

21. *Annual Catalogue and Announcements of the Medical College of Virginia, Richmond:*

Catalogue of Session 1914–1915 and Announcements of Session 1916–1917, Annual Reports, MCVA.

22. University of Louisville Medical Department, *Fifty-eighth Annual Announcement, Session of 1894–95* and *Fifty-fifth Annual Announcement, Session of 1891–92*, Catalogs and Announcements, KHSL.

23. Rothstein, *American Medical Schools*, 134.

24. Membership Records, 1900–1925, WVSMAH.

25. Ibid.

26. Ibid. More than a third of those who did not intern graduated from regional institutions such as the Medical College of Virginia, the University of Louisville, the College of Physicians and Surgeons in Baltimore, Maryland Medical College, the University of Maryland, University College of Medicine in Richmond, and the Baltimore Medical College.

27. Ibid.

28. Ibid.

29. Ibid.

30. Friedson, "Are the Professions Necessary?," 16.

31. Shryock, *Medicine and Society in America*, 148–49; Starr, *Social Transformation of American Medicine*, 57–58.

32. Starr, *Social Transformation of American Medicine*, 90–91.

33. Ibid.

34. Kett, *Formation of the American Medical Profession*, 73.

35. Isaac Carrington Harrison, "A Historical Sketch of the Medical Society of Virginia," *VMM* 59, no. 9 (December 1932): 509–10.

36. Ibid., 510.

37. John W. Kelly, "Kentucky's Contributions to Medicine," *Bulletin of the Kentucky State Department of Health* 15, no. 3 (October 1942): 556.

38. West Virginia State Medical Association, *Transactions*, 8–9.

39. Ibid., 9.

40. C. H. Maxwell, "Pennsylvania and West Virginia Medical Associations: A Comparison," *WVMJ* 2, no. 4 (October 1907): 106–7.

41. "Report of the Business Manager," *KMJ* 9, no. 9 (September 1911): 762.

42. "McDowell County Society," *WVMJ* 7, no. 7 (January 1913): 248.

43. "Clinch Valley Medical Society," *VMM* 55, no. 2 (May 1928): 157.

44. Jones, *Annual Report of the State Department of Mines for the Year Ending December, 1925*, 139; U.S. Department of Commerce, Bureau of the Census, *Fourteenth Census of the United States Taken in the Year 1920*, vol. 1, *Population, 1920*, 107–8.

45. "Report of the Business Manager," *KMJ* 9, no. 9 (September 1911): 762.

46. Ibid., 767–68.

47. John J. Moren, "Report of the Medico-Legal Committee," *KMJ* 9, no. 9 (September 1911): 762.

48. Ibid.; "Report of the Business Manager," *KMJ* 12, no. 9 (September 1914): 555.

49. Kaufmann, *Misadventures of an Appalachian Doctor*, 91.

50. "Chiropractors," *WVMJ* 19, no. 4 (April 1924): 206.

51. "Report of the Business Manager," *KMJ* 12, no. 9 (September 1914): 553.

52. "The Matter of Fees for Life Insurance Examinations," *WVMJ* 2, no. 1 (July 1907): 6.

53. Kegley, *Wythe County*, 106.

54. Polk, *Medical Register*, 1906; "Component Medical Societies," *WVMJ* 1, no. 2 (October 1906): 100; West Virginia State Licensing Registry, 1885–1917, West Virginia State Board of Medicine, Charleston, W.Va.

55. Polk, *Medical Register*, 1906; "Component Medical Societies," *WVMJ* 1, no. 2 (October 1906): 100; West Virginia State Licensing Registry, 1885–1917, West Virginia State Board of Medicine, Charleston, W.Va.

56. Polk, *Medical Register*, 1906; "Component Medical Societies," *WVMJ* 1, no. 2 (October 1906): 100; West Virginia State Licensing Registry, 1885–1917, West Virginia State Board of Medicine, Charleston, W.Va.

57. Starr, *Social Transformation of American Medicine*, 99.

58. Warner, "Ideals of Science," 464.

59. C. B. Williams, "Ten Years Experience in Obstetrics, with Conclusions," *WVMJ* 3, no. 7 (July 1907): 7.

60. S. L. Jepson, "Medical Impostors," *WVMJ* 10, no. 11 (November 1914): 163.

61. E. E. Bickers, "The True Physician," *KMJ* 12, no. 6 (June 1914): 342.

62. R. R. Flannagan, "The Spirit of the Oath," *VMM* 57, no. 8 (November 1930): 541.

63. Leavitt, *Healthiest City*, 78.

64. Ibid., 76–121.

65. Rosenkrantz, "Cart before Horse," 61.

66. "The Early Physicians of the Sandy River District," #92159, CFC.

67. James P. Boggs to State Board of Health, 15 August 1903; W. T. Nolen to State Board of Health, 12 August 1903; W. T. Amyx to State Board of Health, 10 August 1903; M. C. Kash to State Board of Health, 17 August 1903; E. Kelley to State Board of Health, 28 August 1903; and H. H. Stallard to State Board of Health, 31 August 1903, all in General Report of the State Board of Health of Kentucky, 1902–3, WPAHMKC.

68. B. W. Smock to J. N. McCormack, 18 July 1898, General Report of the State Board of Health of Kentucky, 1902–3, WPAHMKC.

69. Lewis, *Transforming the Appalachian Countryside*, 211–34. Lewis examines the conflicts between "new men" and "old men" at the county level during the development of the region.

70. Leavitt, *Healthiest City*, 7.

71. Board of Health of the State of West Virginia, *Biennial Report*, 1908–9, 9–13.

72. *Virginia Health Bulletin* 2, no. 8 (August 1910): 209–11.

73. County Health Officers, 1896–97, Biennial Report of the State Board of Health of Kentucky, WPAHMKC.

74. Rosenkrantz, "Cart before Horse," 61–62; Warner, "Ideals of Science," 464.

75. Friedson, "Are the Professions Necessary?," 16.

76. Numbers, "Rise and Fall of the American Medical Association," 188.

77. Rosen, *History of Public Health*, 324–25. On state-sponsored public health reforms, see Leavitt, *Typhoid Mary*, chap. 2.

78. Felix Swope, "Brief History of the Virginia State Board of Medicine," n.d., Virginia State Board of Medicine, Richmond, Va.

79. Virginia State Medical Examining Board, Minutes, 15 November 1884, "Minutes of Board from Organization in 1884, Together with Results of Examinations from 1884 to December 16–18, 1902," Collection #37, Virginia State Medical Examining Board Records, VSA.

80. Ibid., 15 September 1885, 7 April, 26 October 1886.

81. "The First Century: A History of the Virginia Board of Medical Examiners," unpublished manuscript, Virginia State Board of Medicine, Richmond, Va.

82. Virginia State Medical Examining Board, Minutes, 26 October 1886, "Minutes of Board from Organization in 1884, Together with Results of Examinations from 1884 to December 16–18, 1902," Collection #37, Virginia State Medical Examining Board Records, VSA.

83. Ibid.

84. Bonner, *Becoming a Physician*, 266, 284.

85. "Report of the Business Manager," *KMJ* 9, no. 9 (September 1911): 762. The Kentucky State Medical Society was, by the first decade of the twentieth century, quite strong in the western cities of the state, as the percentage of physicians enrolled in their respective county medical societies demonstrates. The Jefferson County Medical Society attracted 98 percent of Louisville's eligible practitioners. Ninety-three percent of the physicians in Carroll and Trimble Counties allied with the state organization, and all of the area's eligible practitioners joined the Garrard County Medical Society.

86. John W. Kelly, "Kentucky's Contributions to Medicine," *Bulletin of the Kentucky State Department of Health* 15, no. 3 (October 1942): 556.

87. Burrow, *Organized Medicine*, 17.

88. A. Golden, "The Evolution of Medical Legislation in West Virginia," *WVMJ* 12, no. 10 (April 1918): 363.

89. "Laughable or Pitiful, Which?," *WVMJ* 9, no. 1 (January 1915): 240.

90. C. A. Ray, "Report of the Committee on Legislation and Public Policy of the West Virginia State Medical Association," *WVMJ* 21, no. 8 (August 1925): 411.

91. "Cults Again," *WVMJ* 20, no. 6 (June 1925): 317.

92. H. U. Stephenson, "Report of the Legislative Committee," *VMM* 53, no. 1 (April 1926): 56–57.

93. Ibid., 56. In both West Virginia and Virginia, the chiropractors gained strength because a diversity of opinion existed within the medical profession over the merits of chiropracty. A 1924 letter to the editor in the *VMM* argued that the medical association was wrong to attempt to influence the state's attitudes toward sectarian practitioners. The author asserted that perhaps regular physicians should look to their own affairs and "continue to meet scientific standards and continue to raise them as science advances," leaving the problem

of regulating medical practice to the state. See Burnley Lankford, "An Open Letter to the Medical Profession of Virginia," *VMM* 51, no. 1 (April 1924): 49. Other regular physicians argued that doctors might gain constructive instruction from alternative practitioners, a debate reminiscent of the arguments Warner has documented among physicians in New York State in the last decades of the nineteenth century. See J. Allison Hodges, "Shall They Pass?," *VMM* 53, no. 9 (December 1926): 558, and Warner, "Ideals of Science," 462–63.

94. "The Law and the Physician," *WVMJ* 6, no. 9 (March 1912): 314.

95. "Report of the Legislative Committee," *WVMJ* 20, no. 5 (May 1928): 263.

96. Burnley Lankford, "An Open Letter to the Medical Profession of Virginia," *VMM* 51, no. 1 (April 1924): 50.

97. "Chiropractors," *WVMJ* 19, no. 4 (April 1924): 206.

98. J. R. Schultz, "Ethical Silence versus Rational Publicity as a Common Sense Medical Policy," *WVMJ* 20, no. 7 (July 1925): 350.

99. See Osterud, *Bonds of Community*.

100. Borst, *Catching Babies*, 54–67; "Mingo County Register of Physicians and Accoucheurs," Mingo County, West Virginia, Historical Records Survey, microfilm, WVRHC.

101. See Corbin, *Life, Work, and Rebellion*.

102. See Waller, *Feud*.

103. *Logan County Births*, 1872–1900, 1–52.

104. Borst, *Catching Babies*, 61–62.

105. *Logan County Births*, 1872–1900, 1–52; U.S. Department of Commerce, Bureau of the Census, *Tenth Census of the United States*, 1880, and *Twelfth Census of the United States*, 1900, Manuscript Schedule, Logan County, West Virginia, microfilm, WVRHC.

106. *Logan County Births*, 1872–1900, 1–52.

107. The most moving and illustrative depiction of lay midwifery is Laurel Thatcher Ulrich's *Midwife's Tale*. See also Logan, *Motherwit*, and Susie, *In the Ways of Our Grandmothers*. Borst's *Catching Babies* is a unique analytical study of the training of midwives and their rejection of professionalization.

108. U.S. Department of Commerce, Bureau of the Census, *Tenth Census of the United States*, 1880, and *Twelfth Census of the United States*, 1900, Manuscript Schedule, Logan County, West Virginia, Historical Records Survey, microfilm, WVRHC.

109. Ibid.

110. Ibid.

111. Waller, *Feud*, 186.

112. Polk, *Medical and Surgical Directory*, 1886, 940–45.

113. Polk, *Medical and Surgical Register*, 1896, 1523–34.

114. Polk, *Medical Register*, 1917, 1564, 1566.

115. Maggard, "From Farmers to Miners," 35–40; Pudup, "Boundaries of Class," 159.

116. Borst, "Wisconsin's Midwives."

117. Tams, *Smokeless Coal Fields*, 51–53.

118. McGill, *Welfare of Children*, 50.

119. Board of Health of the State of West Virginia, *Biennial Report*, 1930, 11; Bickley, "Midwifery in West Virginia," 56, 64.

120. Belanger, "Midwives' Tales," 44.

121. Ibid.

122. On reciprocity in rural communities, see Borst, *Catching Babies*, 54–67.

123. Annie Veech, "A Practical Solution to Kentucky's Midwife Problem," William Hutchins Papers, SAA.

124. Efird, "Geography of Lay Midwifery," 53.

125. Belanger, "Midwives' Tales," 43–44.

126. Friedson, "Are the Professions Necessary?," 16, 18; Larson, "Production of Expertise," 34.

Chapter Three

1. Skocpol, *Protecting Soldiers and Mothers*, 354; Ladd-Taylor, *Mother-Work*, 32–34; Sklar, "Explaining the Power of Women's Political Culture," 54.

2. Ladd-Taylor, *Mother-Work*, 32, 45; Cott, *Grounding of Modern Feminism*, 91; Tice, "School-Work and Mother-Work," 208.

3. Wertz and Wertz, *Lying-in*, 152–54; Litoff, *American Midwives*, 27; Leavitt, *Brought to Bed*, 201; McMillen, *Motherhood in the Old South*, 183; Hoffert, *Private Matters*, 46.

4. Skocpol, *Protecting Soldiers and Mothers*, 362–67; Skocpol, Abend-Wein, Howard, and Lehmann, "Women's Associations," 696; Anne Firor Scott, *Natural Allies*, 141–58.

5. Skocpol, *Protecting Soldiers and Mothers*, 36.

6. Shaw, "Black Club Women," 16.

7. Hewitt, *Women's Activism and Social Change*, 44.

8. Smith, "Walk-ons in the Third Act," 6.

9. Wells, *Unity in Diversity*, 225.

10. Blair, *Clubwoman as Feminist*, 18; Scott, *Natural Allies*, 2–5.

11. Anne Firor Scott, *Natural Allies*, 126.

12. Wells, *Unity in Diversity*, 74–75, 152–53.

13. Ibid., 471–73.

14. Anne Firor Scott, "After Suffrage," 300.

15. Wells, *Unity in Diversity*, 427; Forderhase, " 'Clear Call of Thoroughbred Women,' " 20.

16. Frances Simrall Riker, "Historical Sketches of Kentucky Federation of Women's Clubs: From Organization, 1894, through Administration ending June, 1909," 1929, Kentucky Federation of Women's Clubs Headquarters, Louisville, Ky.

17. Club History Report, Kentucky, Finding Guides, GFWCWHRC.

18. Harvey, *Silver Gleam*, 55.

19. West Virginia Federation of Women's Clubs, *Yearbook*, 1904–5, 4.

20. Harvey, *Silver Gleam*, 100; "Woman's Club Activities Gain Many Civic Improvements," *Bluefield Daily Telegraph*, 14 December 1939.

21. On the fight over suffrage in Virginia, see Lebsock, "Woman Suffrage and White Supremacy."

22. Anne Firor Scott, *Natural Allies*, 130.

23. "Will Not Join National Body," 15 May 1908, box 1, Meetings Folder, 1907–8, Virginia Federation of Women's Clubs Records, VSA.

24. Mrs. H. M. Dusenberry, "Brief History of the Virginia Federation of Women's Clubs, 1907–1908," Personalities Files, box 1, Virginia Federation of Women's Clubs Records, VSA.

25. Ibid.

26. "Clubs Organized before 1930," box 4, incomplete material, Virginia Federation of Women's Clubs Records, VSA.

27. Mrs. H. M. Dusenberry, "Brief History of the Virginia Federation of Women's Clubs, 1907–1908," Personalities Files, box 1, Virginia Federation of Women's Clubs Records, VSA.

28. Lewis, *Transforming the Appalachian Countryside*, 193–205.

29. Jane Becker, *Selling Tradition*, 45.

30. On the growth of the consumer market, see Lewis, *Transforming the Appalachian Countryside*, 191–93.

31. Callahan, *History of West Virginia*, 3:366.

32. Ibid., 116–17.

33. Ibid., 2:544; "The Women's Club, Beckley, West Virginia, 1917–1918," Pamphlet #4747, Women's Club of Beckley Papers, WVRHC.

34. Callahan, *History of West Virginia*, 2:307.

35. Ibid., 602; "The Women's Club, Beckley, West Virginia, 1914–1915," Pamphlet #4747, Women's Club of Beckley Papers, WVRHC.

36. Callahan, *History of West Virginia*, 2:366–67; "The Women's Club, Beckley, West Virginia, 1914–1915," Pamphlet #4747, Women's Club of Beckley Papers, WVRHC.

37. "Woman's Club Activities Gain Many Civic Improvements," *Bluefield Daily Telegraph*, 14 December 1939.

38. West Virginia Federation of Women's Clubs, *Yearbook*, 1927–28, 24.

39. Harvey, *Silver Gleam*, 100.

40. Polk, *Bluefield, West Virginia, Directory*, 1920–33.

41. "Woman's Club Activities Gain Many Civic Improvements," *Bluefield Daily Telegraph*, 14 December 1939.

42. Polk, *Bluefield, West Virginia, Directory*, 1920–33.

43. Handy, *Social Recorder of Virginia*, 136.

44. Sam T. Mallison, "Mrs. Price Is Interesting Speaker on Child Health," West Virginia Crippled Children, 1936–44, Group IX—General Files, General Class Records, USPHSC.

45. West Virginia Federation of Women's Clubs, *Yearbook*, 1932–33, 84.

46. "The Women's Club of Beckley, West Virginia, 1920–1921," Pamphlet #4747, Women's Club of Beckley Papers, WVRHC.

47. Reid, *West Virginia State Nurses' Association*, 22–23.

48. "The West Virginia Healthfinder," Pamphlet #2153, West Virginia Tuberculosis and Health Association Papers, WVRHC.

49. West Virginia Federation of Women's Clubs, *Manual*, 1910–11, 27.

50. Ehrenreich and English, *For Her Own Good*, 72–73.

51. Ladd-Taylor and Umansky, "*Bad*" *Mothers*, 9.

52. Reid, *West Virginia State Nurses' Association*, 80.

53. Harvey, *Silver Gleam*, 79.

54. Hogshead, *Past Presidents*, 35, 39, 45.

55. Ibid., 13.

56. Callahan, *History of West Virginia*, 2:542–43.

57. Rosenberg, *Care of Strangers*, 346.

58. Leavitt, *Brought to Bed*, 173.

59. "Dr. Mason Combs Hospital, Pineville, 1914," file 105, box 9, and "Harlan Hospital, 1928," file 18, box 10, WPAHMKC.

60. Polk, *Bluefield, West Virginia, Directory*, 1925–26, 798–99.

61. Stuart McGehee, "A Century of Care: A History of Bluefield Regional Medical Center, Bluefield Community Hospital, Bluefield Sanitarium," unpublished manuscript, ERCA.

62. C. Bradley, "Who Pays the Price?," *Mountain Life and Work* 6, no. 3 (October 1930): 9.

63. Leavitt, *Typhoid Mary*, 8; Rosenberg and Vogel, *Therapeutic Revolution*, 39–52.

64. "Program, Division of Health," Department of Public Welfare, file 0709039-1-33, box 2, Winter Program Records, GFWCWHRC.

65. "The Nation's Womanhood Must Defend the Nation's Health," Division of Health, file 0712088-5-3, box 5, Poole Program Records, GFWCWHRC (emphasis in original).

66. "Help Fight the Big Fight," Division of Health, file 0710038-4-18, box 4, Sherman Program Records, GFWCWHRC.

67. "Program, Division of Health," Department of Public Welfare, file 0709039-1-33, box 2, Winter Program Records, GFWCWHRC.

68. "Every Home a Health Center," American Home Department and Public Welfare Department, file 0710092-4-18, box 4, Sherman Program Records, GFWCWHRC.

69. "Program, Division of Health," Department of Public Welfare, file 0709039-1-33, box 2, Winter Program Records, GFWCWHRC.

70. "Program, Division of Child Welfare," Division of Child Welfare, file 0709038-1-32, box 2, Sherman Program Records, GFWCWHRC; "Program, Division of Health," Department of Public Welfare, file 0709039-1-33, box 2, Winter Program Records, GFWCWHRC.

71. Mrs. George P. Boomsliter, "Women's Organizations' Interest in Public Health," *Quarterly Bulletin of the West Virginia Department of Health* 15, no. 1 (January 1928): 14.

72. "Division of Public Health," in West Virginia Federation of Women's Clubs, *Yearbook*, 1922–23, 23.

73. "Federation of Virginia Clubs in Session," *Staunton News Leader*, 31 October 1923.

74. Julia Halsey Harrison, "Special State Work," *Club Life in the Old Dominion* 1, no. 1 (November 1922): 6.

75. Charles Blankenship, Assistant Surgeon General, to Don W. Hatton, Director, Wetzel County Health Department, Cities and Counties File, box 120, USPHSC.

76. "Dr. Stucky Is Heard by a Mixed Audience," *Lexington Herald*, n.d., file 9, box 1, J. A. Stucky Records, SAA.

77. T. W. Moore, "The Betterment of the Medical Profession," *WVMJ* 5, no. 5 (November 1910): 149.

78. "Dr. Stucky Is Heard by a Mixed Audience," *Lexington Herald*, n.d., file 9, box 1, J. A. Stucky Records, SAA.

79. "What the Women's Clubs Can Do," *Quarterly Bulletin of the West Virginia State Board of Health* 2, no. 3 (July 1915): 95.

80. "Prominent Speakers Talk at Woman's Clubs," file 3, box 1, J. A. Stucky Records, SAA.

81. "Co-operation of State Board of Health and Kentucky Women's Clubs," *Bulletin of the State Board of Health of Kentucky* 2, no. 6 (April 1913): 1.

82. Wells, *Unity in Diversity*, 223–24; Ladd-Taylor, *Mother-Work*, 89.

83. Virginia Woodley, "Civics and Public Health," in West Virginia Federation of Women's Clubs, *Yearbook*, 1917–18, 38–40; "The Women's Club of Salem," box 2, Club Histories, Virginia Federation of Women's Clubs Records, VSA; Meckel, *Save the Babies*, 147–48. Meckel finds that middle-class women also participated in baby competitions. Evidence from the coalfields suggests that these contests were typically aimed at working-class Appalachian women.

84. "Report of District Chairmen, First District," in Virginia Federation of Women's Clubs, *Yearbook*, 1929–30, 37–38; Ladd-Taylor and Umansky, *"Bad" Mothers*, 11.

85. "Report of the Southern District," in West Virginia Federation of Women's Clubs, *Yearbook*, 1931–32, 61.

86. "The Woman's Club of Omar," in West Virginia Federation of Women's Clubs, *Yearbook*, 1926–27, 98.

87. Ibid., 98–99.

88. Ibid., 99.

89. "Report of the Southern District," in West Virginia Federation of Women's Clubs, *Yearbook*, 1931–32, 61.

90. Polk, *Bluefield, West Virginia, Directory*, 1920–33.

91. Whisnant, *All That Is Native and Fine*, 19.

92. Sklar, "Hull House in the 1890s," 658–59; Muncy, *Creating a Female Dominion*. For a consideration of the "New Woman" in a broader context, see Fass, *The Damned and the Beautiful*.

93. Forderhase, " 'Clear Call of Thoroughbred Women,' " 28–29.

94. Baker, "Domestication of Politics," 620–21.

95. Breckinridge, *Wide Neighborhoods*, xix.

96. Cornett, "Angel for the Blind," 34.

97. Breckinridge, *Wide Neighborhoods*, 75–77.

98. Muncy, *Creating a Female Dominion*; Tice, "School-Work and Mother-Work," 195–97. For a discussion of the professionalization of women social workers,

see Kunzell, *Fallen Women, Problem Girls*, and Walkowitz, "Making of a Feminine Professional Identity."

99. Jane Becker, *Selling Tradition*, 59.

100. Ibid.

101. Davis, *Spearheads for Reform*, 3–5.

102. Whisnant, *All That Is Native and Fine*, 21–22.

103. Davis, *Spearheads for Reform*, 8–9; Lissak, *Pluralism and Progressives*, 14–15.

104. Whisnant, *All That Is Native and Fine*, 70–71.

105. Quoted in Tice, "School-Work and Mother-Work," 208. On social control in Appalachian settlements, see ibid., 192–93; Whisnant, *All That Is Native and Fine*; and Jane Becker, *Selling Tradition*. For a broader discussion of social control in American settlement and reform movements, see Crocker, *Social Work and Social Order*; Karger, *Sentinels of Order*; Odem, *Delinquent Daughters*; and Rose, "Taking on a Mother's Job."

106. Lucy Furman, "Katherine Pettit, Pioneer Mountain Worker," *Notes from the Pine Mountain Settlement School* 8, no. 1 (November 1936): n.p.

107. Whisnant, *All That Is Native and Fine*, 34.

108. Ibid.

109. Lucy Furman, "Katherine Pettit, Pioneer Mountain Worker," *Notes from the Pine Mountain Settlement School* 8, no. 1 (November 1936): n.p.

110. Ibid.

111. Whisnant, *All That Is Native and Fine*, 34; Lucy Furman, "Katherine Pettit, Pioneer Mountain Worker," *Notes from the Pine Mountain Settlement School* 8, no. 1 (November 1936): n.p.

112. Lucy Furman, "Katherine Pettit, Pioneer Mountain Worker," *Notes from the Pine Mountain Settlement School* 8, no. 1 (November 1936): n.p.

113. Ibid.

114. Tice, "School-Work and Mother-Work," 208–10.

115. Elizabeth Watts to J. A. Stucky, 27 November 1928, file 11, box 1, J. A. Stucky Records, SAA.

116. Elizabeth Peck, "Triumph over Trachoma," *Louisville Courier Journal*, 11 November 1956.

117. J. A. Stucky, "Trachoma: The Scourge of the Mountains," *Southern Mountain Life and Work* 2, no. 3 (October 1926): 3–6.

118. Elizabeth Peck, "Triumph over Trachoma," *Louisville Courier Journal*, 11 November 1956.

119. Isabelle Lyman, "Pioneering against Blindness in the Kentucky Mountains: The Story of Linda Neville," unpublished manuscript, box 1, LNC.

120. Ibid.

121. Ibid.

122. Hortense Flexner, "Fightin' the Blindness," *Red Cross Magazine*, April 1920, box 1, LNC.

123. Isabelle Lyman, "Pioneering against Blindness in the Kentucky Mountains: The Story of Linda Neville," unpublished manuscript, box 1, LNC.

124. "We Are Interested in the Formation of a Kentucky Society for the Prevention of Blindness," 27 May 1910, box 74, LNC.

125. Isabelle Lyman, "Pioneering against Blindness in the Kentucky Mountains: The Story of Linda Neville," unpublished manuscript, box 1, LNC.

126. Linda Neville, "Blindness in Kentucky," *Bulletin of the State Board of Health of Kentucky* 2, no. 6 (April 1913): 26–27.

127. Whisnant, *All That Is Native and Fine*, 38–41.

128. Forderhase, " 'Clear Call of Thoroughbred Women,' " 28.

129. Dye, "Mary Breckinridge," 485–88.

130. Breckinridge, *Wide Neighborhoods*, 159.

131. "Personnel of the Kentucky Committee for Mothers and Babies," *Quarterly Bulletin of the Kentucky Committee for Mothers and Babies* 1, no. 2 (October 1925): 1–3; "We Are Interested in the Formation of a Kentucky Society for the Prevention of Blindness," 27 May 1910, box 74, LNC; "Health Department, Kentucky Federation of Women's Clubs," *Bulletin of the State Board of Health of Kentucky* 1, no. 10 (November 1911): 95.

132. Breckinridge, *Wide Neighborhoods*, 182–83, 194–95.

133. Skocpol, *Protecting Soldiers and Mothers*, 482; Ladd-Taylor, *Mother-Work*, 45.

134. Whisnant, *All That Is Native and Fine*, 12–13; Jane Becker, *Selling Tradition*, 59–61.

135. Isabelle Lyman, "Pioneering against Blindness in the Kentucky Mountains: The Story of Linda Neville," unpublished manuscript, box 1, LNC.

136. Shapiro, *Appalachia on Our Mind*, 142; Batteau, *Invention of Appalachia*, 62–63.

137. J. A. Stucky, "Trachoma: The Scourge of the Mountains," *Southern Mountain Life and Work* 2, no. 3 (October 1926): 5.

138. Whisnant, *All That Is Native and Fine*, 57–58.

139. Jane Becker, *Selling Tradition*, 77–78.

140. J. A. Stucky, "Thousands in Mountains of Kentucky Are Pleading for Opportunity to Learn," 30 September 1923, file 7, box 7, J. A. Stucky Records, SAA; Hortense Flexner, "Fightin' the Blindness," *Red Cross Magazine*, April 1920, box 1, LNC; Tice, "Mother-Work and School-Work," 208–9.

Chapter Four

1. Muncy, *Creating a Female Dominion*, 135–43.

2. Reverby, *Ordered to Care*, 129; Buhler-Wilkerson, *False Dawn*, 92.

3. Flanagan, "Gender and Urban Political Reform," 1046, 1047–48.

4. Edith Abbot, quoted in Ladd-Taylor, *Mother-Work*, 78.

5. Sklar, "Historical Foundations of Women's Power," 69.

6. Armeny, "Organized Nurses," 16.

7. Koven and Michel, "Womanly Duties," 1077.

8. Ladd-Taylor, " 'Grannies' and 'Spinsters,' " 260–63.

9. Brickman, "Public Health, Midwives, and Nurses," 72, 74, 79.

10. Sklar, "Hull House Maps and Papers," 117.

11. Ibid., 116.

12. Lydia Roberts, *Nutrition and Care of Children*; McGill, *Welfare of Children*.

13. Mary Breckinridge, "Midwifery in the Kentucky Mountains: An Investigation," 1923, unpublished manuscript, MIKL.

14. W. Bertram Ireland, "Safeguarding Mothers and Babies in the Highlands," 1926, box 72, LNC; Willeford, "Income and Health," 21.

15. "Community Health Study Outline," file 0712088-5-1, box 5, Poole Program Records, GFWCWHRC.

16. Jean T. Dillon, "Report of Public Health Division," in West Virginia Federation of Women's Clubs, *Yearbook*, 1923–24, 69–70.

17. Margaret P. Kuyk, "Report of Chairman of Health," in Virginia Federation of Women's Clubs, *Yearbook*, 1923–24, 61–62.

18. Ladd-Taylor, "Toward Defining Maternalism," 111.

19. McGill, *Welfare of Children*, 11, 13, 14–15, 48–49.

20. Frankel and Dublin, *Sickness among Coal Miners*, 13–14.

21. McGill, *Welfare of Children*, 49.

22. U.S. Coal Commission, *Report of the United States Coal Commission, Part III*, 1495.

23. Ibid., 1503–27.

24. Mary Breckinridge, "Midwifery in the Kentucky Mountains: An Investigation," 1923, unpublished manuscript, MIKL.

25. W. Bertram Ireland, "Safeguarding Mothers and Babies in the Highlands," 1926, box 72, LNC, 10.

26. Sklar, "Historical Foundations of Women's Power," 69.

27. Ladd-Taylor and Umansky, *"Bad" Mothers*, 9.

28. Corbin, *Life, Work, and Rebellion*, 135.

29. Ploss, "History of the Medical Care Program," 18.

30. McGill, *Welfare of Children*, 49.

31. Mrs. Andrew Wilson, "Public Welfare," in West Virginia Federation of Women's Clubs, *Yearbook*, 1922–23, 169.

32. Jean Dillon, "Division of Child Welfare," in West Virginia Federation of Women's Clubs, *Yearbook*, 1922–23, 137–38.

33. "Public Welfare," in West Virginia Federation of Women's Clubs, *Yearbook*, 1923–24, 41.

34. "Public Health," in Virginia Federation of Women's Clubs, *Yearbook*, 1911–12, 12.

35. "Report of Division of Public Welfare," in West Virginia Federation of Women's Clubs, *Yearbook*, 1920–21, 36.

36. Haury Davily, "Owingsville Woman's Club," *KMJ* 23, no. 3 (March 1924): 99.

37. "Public Welfare," in Virginia Federation of Women's Clubs, *Yearbook*, 1929–30, 89.

38. Mrs. Andrew Wilson, "Division of Public Welfare," in West Virginia Federation of Women's Clubs, *Yearbook*, 1922–23, 138.

39. "The Prestonsburg Woman's Club," file 1301-20-14, box 20, Club Histories Collection, GFWCWHRC.

40. Rothman, *Woman's Proper Place*, 137–38.

41. Jean Dillon, "Department of Public Welfare," *West Virginia Clubwoman* 3, no. 3 (February 1924): n.p.; Mrs. Andrew Wilson, "Division of Public Health," in West Virginia Federation of Women's Clubs, *Yearbook*, 1922–23, 139.

42. "Woman's Club Work," *KMJ* 9, no. 6 (June 1911): 461.

43. "Mortality High in Mingo Figures Show," *Williamson Daily News*, 23 December 1923, 1; Barney, "Health Services," 47.

44. See General Reports of the State Board of Health of Kentucky, file 11, box 67, WPAHMKC.

45. Barney, "Health Services," 47.

46. Buhler-Wilkerson, *False Dawn*, ix; Armeny, "Organized Nurses," 14.

47. Mrs. George DeBolt, "Department of Public Welfare," *West Virginia Clubwoman* 2, no. 3 (February 1923): n.p.

48. Mrs. Andrew Wilson, "Public Welfare," in West Virginia Federation of Women's Clubs, *Yearbook*, 1922–23, 169.

49. Mrs. George DeBolt, "Department of Public Welfare," *West Virginia Clubwoman* 2, no. 3 (February 1923): n.p.

50. Buhler-Wilkerson, *False Dawn*, 92; Armeny, "Organized Nurses," 14; Melosh, "*Physician's Hand*," 114, 122.

51. Melosh, "*Physician's Hand*," 113.

52. Buhler-Wilkerson, *False Dawn*, ix.

53. "Report of Department of Public Welfare," in West Virginia Federation of Women's Clubs, *Yearbook*, 1917–18, 31; "History of Radford Woman's Club," box 2, Club Histories, Virginia Federation of Women's Clubs Records, VSA.

54. *West Virginia Healthfinder*, May 1926, A&M #2357, West Virginia Tuberculosis and Health Association Papers, WVRHC.

55. Buhler-Wilkerson, *False Dawn*, 90.

56. "Report of Department of Public Welfare," in West Virginia Federation of Women's Clubs, *Yearbook*, 1925–26, 88.

57. "Report of Bramwell Woman's Club," *West Virginia Clubwoman* 3, no. 7 (October 1924): n.p.

58. "Report of Radford Woman's Club," *Virginia Clubwoman* 1, no. 3 (January–February 1929): 11.

59. Ladd-Taylor and Umansky, "*Bad*" *Mothers*, 11–12.

60. Melosh, "*Physician's Hand*," 139.

61. Gazelle Hundley Hume, "Report of the Division of Public Health," West Virginia Federation of Women's Clubs, *Yearbook*, 1932–33, 84.

62. "The Federation Clinic," *Virginia Clubwoman* 8, no. 2 (November 1931): 5.

63. Ransom, "Bureau of Public Health Nursing," 83.

64. "Report of Division of Public Health," in West Virginia Federation of Women's Clubs, *Yearbook*, 1924–25, 56.

65. "Southern District Meeting," in West Virginia Federation of Women's Clubs, *Yearbook*, 1922–23, 94.

66. "Annual Report of Department of Public Welfare," in West Virginia Federation of Women's Clubs, *Yearbook*, 1921–22, 98.

67. Jean Dillon, "Department of Public Welfare," *West Virginia Clubwoman* 3,

no. 3 (February 1924): n.p.; *West Virginia Healthfinder*, January–February 1921, A&M #2357, West Virginia Tuberculosis and Health Association Papers, WVRHC.

68. "Report of the Southern District," in West Virginia Federation of Women's Clubs, *Yearbook*, 1932–33, 68.

69. Reverby, *Ordered to Care*; Melosh, *"Physician's Hand,"* 114.

70. Reverby, *Ordered to Care*, 110.

71. Virginia Woodley, "Civics and Public Health," in West Virginia Federation of Women's Clubs, *Yearbook*, 1917–18, 39.

72. Linda Neville, "A Case of Ophthalmia Neonatorum in a Remote Isolated Place in Kentucky," 1916, box 1A, LNC.

73. "The Woman's Club of Salem," box 2, Club Histories, Virginia Federation of Women's Clubs Records, VSA.

74. "Report of Department of Public Health," in West Virginia Federation of Women's Clubs, *Yearbook*, 1920–21, 60.

75. "Report of Division of Public Health," in West Virginia Federation of Women's Clubs, *Yearbook*, 1919–20, 78.

76. "Division of Health," Department of Public Welfare, file 0710037-4-10, box 4, Sherman Program Records, GFWCWHRC.

77. "Public Health in Americanization Plans," Department of Public Welfare, file 0709047-1-38, box 2, Winter Program Records, GFWCWHRC.

78. Melosh, *"Physician's Hand,"* 135.

79. For additional information on the Americanization work of West Virginia clubwomen, see Hennen, *Americanization of West Virginia*, 119–35.

80. "Public Health in Americanization Plans," Department of Public Welfare, file 0709047-1-38, box 2, Winter Program Records, GFWCWHRC.

81. Sam T. Mallison, "Mrs. Price Is Interesting Speaker on Child Health," West Virginia Crippled Children, 1936–44, Group IX—General Files, General Class Records, USPHSC.

82. "Minutes of the Capital District Meeting, May 9, 1922," in West Virginia Federation of Women's Clubs, *Yearbook*, 1922–23, 89.

83. Mrs. G. O. Nagle, "Report of Health Committee," in West Virginia Federation of Women's Clubs, *Manual*, 1908–9.

84. Margaret Kuyk, "Virginia Federation of Women's Clubs," in Virginia Federation of Women's Clubs, *Yearbook*, 1924–25, 61.

85. "Division of Child Hygiene," in Board of Health of the State of West Virginia, *Biennial Report*, 1921–22, 47.

86. Jean Dillon, "Report of Public Health Division," in West Virginia Federation of Women's Clubs, *Yearbook*, 1923–24, 69.

87. "Your Public Policy," *WVMJ* 22, no. 11 (November 1926): 591.

88. Armeny, "Organized Nurses," 15.

89. Rothman describes Margaret Sanger's reliance on medical doctors as a similar effort to achieve advances for women through men's advocacy in *Woman's Proper Place*, 201.

90. Mary Breckinridge, "Midwifery in the Kentucky Mountains: An Investigation," 1923, unpublished manuscript, MIKL.

91. Ibid.

92. Caffin and Caffin, "Experiences of the Nurse-Midwife," 2–3; "County Organization," *Quarterly Bulletin of the Kentucky Committee for Mothers and Babies* 1, no. 2 (October 1925): 4.

93. Mary Breckinridge to William J. Hutchinson, 17 May 1934, file 3, box 1, Frontier Nursing Service Records, SAA.

94. Dye, "Mary Breckinridge," 495.

95. Thomas, *Dawn Comes to the Mountains*, 51.

96. Stucky, "Trachoma among the Natives of the Mountains of Eastern Kentucky," 521.

97. "Thousands in Mountains of Kentucky Are Pleading for Opportunity to Learn," 30 September 1923, file 2, box 3, J. A. Stucky Records, SAA.

98. Borst, *Catching Babies*, 119, 126–29.

99. Glyn A. Morris to Friend, 28 March 1934, file 2, box 2, Pine Mountain Settlement School Records, SAA.

100. Higginbotham, "From Our Mountain Nurses," 28.

101. Mary Breckinridge, "Midwifery in the Kentucky Mountains: An Investigation," 1923, unpublished manuscript, MIKL; Boston Women's Health Book Collective, *Our Bodies, Ourselves*, 446.

102. Ida Stapleton, "The Cabin," June 1927, file 7, box 2, Pine Mountain Settlement School Records, SAA.

103. Ibid.

104. Mary Breckinridge, "Midwifery in the Kentucky Mountains: An Investigation," 1923, unpublished manuscript, MIKL.

105. Ida Stapleton to Friends, 14 December 1926, file 7, box 2 (part 1), Pine Mountain Settlement School Records, SAA.

106. Higginbotham, "Pages from a Diary," 28.

107. "Trachoma Proclamation," box 29, LNC.

108. "Minutes of the House of Delegates," *KMJ* 9, no. 11 (November 1911): 933.

109. Ibid., 934.

110. "Dream Houses," box 74, LNC.

111. Ibid.

112. Flanagan, "Gender and Urban Political Reform," 1046.

113. Rothman, *Woman's Proper Place*, 138–40.

Chapter Five

1. Meckel, *Save the Babies*, 217; Friedson, "Are the Professions Necessary?," 21; Larson, *Rise of Professionalism*, 236.

2. Flanagan, "Gender and Urban Political Reform," 1048.

3. Rothman, "Women's Clinics or Doctors' Offices," 187–88.

4. Starr, *Social Transformation of American Medicine*, 193–94.

5. Leavitt, *Typhoid Mary*, 26; Leavitt, *Healthiest City*, 82–83; Meckel, *Save the Babies*, 100.

6. Ladd-Taylor, *Mother-Work*, 188–89.

7. Quoted in ibid., 188; Rothman, *Woman's Proper Place*, 142; Skocpol, *Protecting Soldiers and Mothers*, 515.

8. Cott, *Grounding of Modern Feminism*, chap. 5.

9. "Minutes of Annual Meeting," *KMJ* 28, no. 2 (February 1930): 80; "Doctors Disapprove Children's Clinic," Mrs. W. F. Moreland File, 1926–28, box 1, Virginia Federation of Women's Clubs Records, VSA.

10. J. A. Stucky to May Stone, 22 July 1912, file 2, box 1, J. A. Stucky Records, SAA.

11. J. A. Stucky to Harriet Butler, 23 August 1911, file 2, box 1, J. A. Stucky Records, SAA.

12. "Announcement," file 3, box 2, J. A. Stucky Records, SAA.

13. Glyn Morris to Friend, 28 March 1934, file 7, box 2, Pine Mountain Settlement School Records, SAA.

14. Caffin and Caffin, "Experiences of the Nurse-Midwife," 3.

15. Anne Firor Scott, *Natural Allies*, 126–27; Koven and Michel, "Womanly Duties," 1091.

16. Vera Andrew Harvey, "State President's Message," in West Virginia Federation of Women's Clubs, *Yearbook*, 1932–33, 7.

17. Rothman discusses the process by which physicians assumed responsibility for preventive health examinations in the 1920s in *Woman's Proper Place*, 144–45. Meckel has enriched that discussion with his examination of changes in medical education and the reconstruction of medical practice during the 1920s in *Save the Babies*, 216–17.

18. "Health Insurance—The Real Kind," *Virginia Health Bulletin* 8, no. 4 (April 1916): 3.

19. Harry Hall, "Agencies That Would Clip the Wings of Medical Progress," *WVMJ* 21, no. 10 (October 1925): 514; Leavitt, *Healthiest City*, 74–75, 200–201.

20. Harry Hall, "Agencies That Would Clip the Wings of Medical Progress," *WVMJ* 21, no. 10 (October 1925): 514.

21. See Numbers, *Almost Persuaded*.

22. W. W. Kerns, "Why Young Physicians Are Not Locating in the Country," *VMM* 54, no. 6 (September 1927): 369.

23. Ibid.

24. Elkins and Young, *Public Health Administration*, 5.

25. "Full Health Unit Aired in Meeting Here," *New Dominion*, 1 August 1929.

26. Clarence Meadows, Attorney General of the State of West Virginia, to Thomas Parran, Surgeon General of the United States, 29 June 1939, file 1616-L, box 119, USPHSC. On physicians' anxiety about socialism in compulsory insurance, see Numbers, *Almost Persuaded*, 77, 88, 110.

27. "Full Health Unit Aired in Meeting Here," *New Dominion*, 1 August 1929.

28. "Dr. Lemley to Explain Full Health Unit," *New Dominion*, 31 July 1929.

29. "Editorial," *New Dominion*, 7 August 1929.

30. "Legislative Committee Report," 13 August 1929, Monongalia County

Medical Society Collection, Closed Collection, Health Sciences Library, West Virginia University, Morgantown, W.Va.

31. "Editorial," *New Dominion*, 2 August 1929.

32. Ibid., 7 August 1929.

33. "County Court Authorizes Full Time Health Unit Here," *New Dominion*, 14 August 1929.

34. The inherent contradiction between women's public activity based on domestic accomplishments and their lack of professional status is explored in Koven and Michel, *Mothers of a New World*, 6–7, 18.

35. Charles S. Webb, "An Open Letter to the Medical Profession of Virginia," *VMM* 57, no. 3 (June 1930): 265.

36. B. B. Bagby, "Deaths from Diphtheria Directly Proportional to Percentage of Immunization," *VMM* 61, no. 2 (May 1934): 108–10.

37. E. G. Williams, "The Debatable Fields of Public Health Activity," *VMM* 53, no. 10 (January 1927): 646.

38. "Doctors Disapprove Children's Clinic," 1927, Mrs. W. F. Moreland File, 1926–28, Virginia Federation of Women's Clubs Records, VSA.

39. E. G. Williams, "The Debatable Fields of Public Health Activity," *VMM* 53, no. 10 (January 1927): 646.

40. "Some Urgent Professional Problems and Their Solutions," *VMM* 57, no. 12 (March 1931): 828.

41. "Eye, Ear, Nose, and Throat Treatment at Big Creek, Clay County, Ky.," September 1923, box 24, LNC.

42. Leavitt, *Healthiest City*, 200–201.

43. "Minutes of Annual Meeting," *KMJ* 28, no. 2 (February 1930): 81.

44. Ennion G. Williams, "Dr. Williams Discusses Attitude of State Department of Health to Curative Clinics," *VMM* 56, no. 3 (June 1929): 199.

45. "Logan County Experiments with Oil," *West Virginia Healthfinder*, January–April 1929, A&M #2357, West Virginia Tuberculosis and Health Association Papers, WVRHC.

46. "Dr. Vest Holds Clinic in Mingo County," *West Virginia Healthfinder*, January–February 1930, A&M #2357, West Virginia Tuberculosis and Health Association Papers, WVRHC.

47. Harriet Butler to J. N. McCormack, 8 November 1911, box 29, LNC.

48. Ibid.

49. Ladd-Taylor, " 'Grannies' and 'Spinsters,' " 255–57; Ladd-Taylor, *Mother-Work*, 188–90; Muncy, *Creating a Female Dominion*, 167.

50. On infant nutrition, see Apple, *Mothers and Medicine*.

51. "Lactic Acid Milk," *WVMJ* 22, no. 1 (January 1926): n.p.

52. "More Significant Now Than Ever Before: The Mead Policy," *VMM* 61, no. 2 (May 1934): n.p.

53. "Curiosity Gave the World a New and Important Medicine . . . Physiological Standardization Made This Medicine Uniformly Potent," *WVMJ* 32, no. 1 (January 1931): iii.

54. Melosh, *"Physician's Hand,"* 146–47.

55. Kobrin, "American Midwife Controversy"; Borst, *Catching Babies*, 117–30.

56. Rushing, "Market Explanations for Occupational Power," 13.

57. Ladd-Taylor, " 'Grannies' and 'Spinsters,' " 256.

58. Brickman, "Public Health, Midwives, and Nurses," 76; E. R. Hardin, "The Midwife Problem," *Southern Medical Journal* 18, no. 5 (May 1925): 347.

59. Walter Edmond Levy, "Our Midwife Problems," *Southern Medical Journal* 24, no. 9 (September 1931): 820.

60. "Your Public Policy," *WVMJ* 22, no. 11 (November 1926): 591.

61. Dye, "Mary Breckinridge," 485.

62. Ibid., 496.

63. Ransom, "Bureau of Public Health Nursing," 81; Melosh, "*Physician's Hand*," 127.

64. Skocpol, *Protecting Soldiers and Mothers*, 482.

65. Jean Dillon to Blanche Haines and Blanche Haines to Jean Dillon, n.d., file 11-50-2 through 11-52-8, Central File, 1925–28, box 342, Children's Bureau Collection, RG 102, NARA.

66. Jean Dillon to Blanche Haines, n.d., file 11-52-2, Official Correspondence, 1925–28, box 342, Children's Bureau Collection, RG 102, NARA.

67. Richard Thrush, "Report of Visit to the State Department of Health, Charleston, West Virginia, January 21, 1927," file 509.2, box 573, Red Cross Collection, RG 200, NARA.

68. Julia Groscop, "Meeting of the Public Health Association and Health Commissioners, November 27–28, 1928," file 509.2, box 573, Red Cross Collection, RG 200, NARA.

69. For a discussion of the professional aspirations of public health nurses, see Buhler-Wilkerson, *False Dawn*; Melosh, "*Physician's Hand*"; and Reverby, *Ordered to Care*.

70. Beard, *Nurse in Public Health*, 7–8.

71. Melosh, "*Physician's Hand*," 143; Reverby, *Ordered to Care*, 130–31.

72. Buhler-Wilkerson, *False Dawn*, ix–xi; Melosh, "*Physician's Hand*," 129.

73. Dr. David Littlejohn to C. E. Waller, Assistant Surgeon General of the United States, 25 May 1933, file 0110-0225, box 73, USPHSC.

74. "Minutes of Business Meetings, 1920–1945," 3 May 1921, Monongalia County Medical Society, Closed Collection, Health Sciences Library, West Virginia University, Morgantown, W.Va.

75. "Proceedings of the Eighteenth Annual Convention of the West Virginia State Nurses' Association, 1924," MS #79-220, box 6, West Virginia State Nurses' Association Records, West Virginia State Archives and Cultural Center, Charleston, W.Va.

76. Reid, *West Virginia State Nurses' Association*, 72.

77. Dillon's reports for the yearbooks of the West Virginia Federation of Women's Clubs were notoriously short. One cannot help but compare them to the much longer and more verbose offerings of other clubwomen who did not undertake professional or public activity beyond the voluntary sphere. See West Virginia Federation of Women's Clubs, *Yearbook* and *West Virginia Clubwoman*, 1911–22.

78. "Proceedings of the Eighteenth Annual Convention of the West Virginia

State Nurses' Association," MS #79-220, box 6, West Virginia State Nurses' Association Records, West Virginia State Archives and Cultural Center, Charleston, W.Va.

79. Richard Thrush, "Report of Visit to the State Department of Health, Charleston, West Virginia, January 21, 1927," and Julia Groscop, "Meeting of the Public Health Association and Health Commissioners, November 27–28, 1928," both in file 509.2, box 573, Red Cross Collection, RG 200, NARA.

80. Mary Keith Cauthern to Annabell Peterson, 25 November 1933, and Julia Groscop, "Report of Visit to State Department of Public Health, February 25–27, 1929," both in file 509.22, box 573, Red Cross Collection, RG 200, NARA. Leavitt chronicles a similar manipulation in Milwaukee in *Healthiest City*, 224. In that case, however, the offending agent was a male sociologist who was replaced by a physician.

81. Reverby, *Ordered to Care*, 130–31, 159, 168–76; Melosh, *"Physician's Hand,"* 39–40.

82. Kathryn Trent, "Comments on Senate Bill," *Weather Vane* 3, no. 2 (September 1929): n.p.

83. Frances Helen Zeigler, "Address over WRVA," *Bits of News from Headquarters, Graduate Nurses' Association of Virginia* 4, no. 1 (April 1936): 12–14.

84. Frances Helen Zeigler, "Bits of News," *Bits of News from Headquarters, Graduate Nurses' Association of Virginia* 4, no. 1 (April 1936): 3–9; Reverby, *Ordered to Care*, 168–76.

85. Rothman, *Woman's Proper Place*, 177–78, 184–87; Cott, *Grounding of Modern Feminism*, 145–74.

86. Mrs. Walter Paxton, "Public Welfare," *Bulletin of the Virginia Federation of Women's Clubs*, n.d., Publications File, box 2, Virginia Federation of Women's Clubs Records, VSA.

87. Mrs. Andrew Wilson, "Report of Public Health Department," in West Virginia Federation of Women's Clubs, *Yearbook*, 1919–20, 76–77.

88. "Sweetmeats, Hams, and Cash Given to Tent Colonists" and "McDowell Responds to Appeal for Relief," *Williamson Daily News*, 23 December 1920; "Mortality Rate High in Mingo Figures Show," *Williamson Daily News*, 24 December 1920.

89. See Corbin, *Life, Work, and Rebellion*; Savage, *Thunder in the Mountains*.

90. "Resolutions," in West Virginia Federation of Women's Clubs, *Yearbook*, 1921–22, 51–52.

91. Ibid.

92. Whites, "De Graffenreid Controversy," 449–50.

93. "A Brief History of the Tazewell Woman's Club," General Histories File, box 4, Virginia Federation of Women's Clubs Records, VSA.

94. Hennen, *Americanization of West Virginia*, 97, 119, 122, 125.

95. Mrs. A. L. Lehman, "Department of Americanization," in West Virginia Federation of Women's Clubs, *Yearbook*, 1921–22, 103–4.

96. Hennen, *Americanization of West Virginia*, 9, 125.

97. Rothman, *Woman's Proper Place*, 187.

98. Jesse D. Hamer, *History of the Woman's Auxiliary to the American Medical Association*, 1922–1952 (n.p., n.d.), Women's Auxiliary of the West Virginia State Medical Association Records, WVSMAH.

99. Mrs. Herbert Ulrich, *Right Side of the Caduceus*, 3.

100. Ibid.

101. Ibid., 5.

102. Hogshead, *Past Presidents*, 13.

103. Mrs. J. T. Reddick, "Report to the House of Delegates, Kentucky State Medical Association," *KMJ* 28, no. 1 (January 1930): 40.

104. "To the Doctors," *VMM* 54, no. 7 (October 1927): 421.

105. Women's Auxiliary of the Medical Society of Virginia, "New Opportunities," *VMM* 57, no. 12 (March 1931): 823.

106. "Minutes of the Fifth Annual Meeting of the Women's Auxiliary to the West Virginia State Medical Association," 21 May 1929, Women's Auxiliary of the West Virginia State Medical Association Records, WVSMAH.

107. "Pre-Convention Executive Board Meeting of the Women's Auxiliary to the West Virginia State Medical Association," 11 July 1938, Women's Auxiliary of the West Virginia State Medical Association Records, WVSMAH.

108. Alice Leigh, "An Appeal for Virginia," *VMM* 55, no. 1 (April 1928): 63.

109. Mrs. F. P. Gengenbach, "Why I Am a Member of the Auxiliary," *VMM* 54, no. 4 (July 1927): 254.

110. "The Auxiliary's Task in Health Education," *VMM* 55, no. 12 (March 1929): 895.

111. "Advantages of Organized Effort among the Women," *VMM* 53, no. 4 (July 1926): 265.

112. "The Auxiliary," *KMJ* 28, no. 10 (October 1930): 472.

113. A. T. McCormack, "Report of Councilor, Eleventh District," *KMJ* 28, no. 11 (November 1930): 525.

114. "Executive Board Meeting of Women's Auxiliary to the West Virginia State Medical Association," 30 September 1932, Women's Auxiliary of the West Virginia State Medical Association Records, WVSMAH.

115. Jesse D. Hamer, *History of the Woman's Auxiliary to the American Medical Association*, 1922–1952 (n.p., n.d.), Women's Auxiliary of the West Virginia State Medical Association Records, WVSMAH.

116. "Health Education through Women's Clubs," *VMM* 54, no. 6 (September 1927): 388–89.

117. "Official Health Program of the Woman's Auxiliary of the American Medical Association," *VMM* 56, no. 10 (February 1930): 767–68.

118. "Program of the Auxiliary," *VMM* 54, no. 12 (March 1928): 803 (emphasis in original).

119. "WLAP Radio Program for First 9 Months," *KMJ* 28, no. 12 (December 1930): 638.

120. "Report of the Letcher County Medical Society," *KMJ* 28, no. 6 (June 1930): 312.

121. "Woman's Auxiliary Notes," *KMJ* 28, no. 2 (February 1928): 122.

122. "Perry County Leads," *KMJ* 28, no. 5 (May 1930): 263.

123. "Report of Committee on Woman's Auxiliary," *KMJ* 28, no. 11 (November 1930): 543.

124. Mrs. J. Newton Hunsberger, "The Questions: Who and Why?," *KMJ* 28, no. 12 (December 1930): 620.

125. "Minutes of Third Annual Meeting of Women's Auxiliary of the West Virginia State Medical Association," 21 June 1927, Women's Auxiliary of the West Virginia State Medical Association Records, WVSMAH.

126. "Warned against Propaganda," *VMM* 55, no. 4 (July 1928): 279–80.

127. "A Letter to the County Chairman of Health Education," *VMM* 56, no. 3 (June 1929): 200–201.

128. Skocpol, *Protecting Soldiers and Mothers*, 515; Rothman, *Woman's Proper Place*, 142.

Conclusion

1. Sklar, "Historical Foundations of Women's Power"; Koven and Michel, *Mothers of a New World*, 1–42; Skocpol, *Protecting Soldiers and Mothers*, 37, 318, 371–72; Evans and Boyte, *Free Spaces*. Skocpol expresses disagreement with Koven and Michel, but she, too, comments on the weakness of the federal bureaucracy at the beginning of Progressive Era benevolence campaigns.

2. Ladd-Taylor and Umansky, *"Bad" Mothers*, 9; Koven and Michel, "Womanly Duties," 1078.

3. Cott, *Grounding of Modern Feminism*, chap. 5.

4. Rothman, *Woman's Proper Place*, 142–43.

5. Skocpol, *Protecting Soldiers and Mothers*, 523–24.

6. "The New Year," *WVMJ* 30, no. 1 (January 1934): 43; Roy Ben Miller, "'President' Page," *WVMJ* 30, no. 6 (June 1934): 244; Starr, *Social Transformation of American Medicine*, 260–72; Rosen, *Structure of American Medical Practice*, 114–15.

7. For an evaluation of the power of the UMWA, see Gaventa, *Power and Powerlessness*.

8. U.S. Department of the Interior, Coal Mines Administration, *Medical Survey of the Bituminous Coal Industry*, vii.

9. Mulcahy, "Health Care in the Coal Fields," 644; Huff, "Effects of the UMWA upon the Reform of the Company Doctor System."

10. Mulcahy, "New Deal for the Coal Miners."

11. Mulcahy, "Health Care in the Coal Fields," 643–45.

12. Ibid., 648, 654.

13. Couto, "Poverty, Politics, and Health Care," 317.

14. Couto, "Political Economy of Appalachian Health," 12; Smith, *Digging Our Own Graves*.

15. Couto, "Appalachian Health Innovations," 170–71.

16. Couto, "Political Economy of Appalachian Health," 5–6.

17. Couto, "Appalachian Health Innovations," 174; Peddle, "To Do What's Right."

18. See Smith, *Digging Our Own Graves*; Cirillo, "Every Mountain Hollow," 4–16; and Couto, "Appalachian Health Innovations," 174.

19. Couto, "Appalachian Health Innovations," 180–81, 183.

20. Doyal and Pennell, *Political Economy of Health*, 43.

21. Peddle, "To Do What's Right."

22. "Midwife License Bill Squeaks by House Tuesday," *West Virginia University Daily Athenaeum*, 12 February 1992.

23. Dawn Miller, "Staying Home to Have the Baby," *Charleston Gazette*, 5 April 1992.

24. Ibid.

25. "License Midwives," *Charleston Gazette*, 16 February 1992.

26. Dawn Miller, "State's Midwives Back Licensing Board Bill," *Charleston Gazette*, 1 February 1992.

27. Fanny Seller, "Midwife Licensing Bill Clears House," *Charleston Gazette*, 12 February 1992.

28. Ibid.

29. Dawn Miller, "Staying Home to Have the Baby," *Charleston Gazette*, 5 April 1992.

30. Skocpol, *Protecting Soldiers and Mothers*, 538.

BIBLIOGRAPHY

Primary Sources

Manuscript Collections

Berea, Kentucky
    Southern Appalachian Archives, Hutchins Library, Berea College
        Council of the Southern Mountains Records
        Frontier Nursing Service Records
        William Hutchins Papers
        Pine Mountain Settlement School Records
        J. A. Stucky Records
Bluefield, West Virginia
    Eastern Regional Coal Archives, Craft Memorial Library
        Bluefield Sanitorium Records
        Foster Collection
        Claude Frazier Collection
Charleston, West Virginia
    West Virginia State Archives and Cultural Center
        West Virginia State Nurses' Association Records
    West Virginia State Board of Medicine
        West Virginia State Licensing Registry, 1885–1917
    West Virginia State Medical Association Headquarters
        Membership Records, 1900–1925
        Women's Auxiliary of the West Virginia State Medical Association
            Records
Frankfort, Kentucky
    Kentucky State Department of Libraries and Archives
        Applications for Medical Licenses, 1890–1925
        Various County Records
Lexington, Kentucky
    Special Collections, M. I. King Library, University of Kentucky
        Frontier Nursing Service Collection
        Linda Neville Collection
Louisville, Kentucky
    Kentucky Federation of Women's Clubs Headquarters
    Kornhauser Health Sciences Library, University of Louisville
        Catalogs and Announcements

Works Progress Administration History of Medicine in Kentucky
Collection
Kentucky State Register of Physicians
Morgantown, West Virginia
Monongalia County Medical Society Collection, Closed Collection, Health
Sciences Library, West Virginia University
West Virginia and Regional History Collection, West Virginia University
Henry D. Hatfield Collection
West Virginia Society of Osteopathic Medicine Records, Pamphlet
Collection
West Virginia Tuberculosis and Health Association Papers
Women's Club of Beckley Papers
Richmond, Virginia
Medical College of Virginia Archives, Tompkins-McCaw Library
Annual Reports, 1914–20
Matriculation Book, 1838–71
Minute Books
Sanger Historical Collection
Virginia State Archives
Virginia Federation of Women's Clubs Records
Virginia State Department of Health Collection
Virginia State Department of Health Regulatory Boards Collection
Virginia State Medical Examining Board Records
Virginia Women's Cultural History Project Records
Virginia State Board of Medicine
Medical Registrations, 1890–1930
Washington, D.C.
General Federation of Women's Clubs Women's History and Resource
Center
Club Histories Collection
General Federation of Women's Clubs Papers
Presidents' Records, Program Records, and State Club Histories, 1898–
1936
National Archives and Records Administration
Children's Bureau Collection, Record Group 102
Red Cross Collection, Record Group 200
U.S. Public Health Service Collection, Record Group 90

Published Works and Dissertations

American Friends Service Committee. *Report of the Child Relief Work in the
Bituminous Coal Fields, September 1, 1931–August 31, 1932.* Philadelphia: Engle,
1932.
Beard, Mary. *The Nurse in Public Health.* New York: Harper and Brothers, 1929.
Brainard, Annie. *Organization of Public Health Nursing.* New York: Macmillan, 1919.

Breckinridge, Mary. *Wide Neighborhoods: A Story of the Frontier Nursing Service*. 1952. Reprint, Lexington: University Press of Kentucky, 1981.

Butler, Samuel. *The Medical Register and Directory of the United States*. Philadelphia: Office of Medical and Surgical Reporter, 1874.

Caffin, Freda, and Caroline Caffin. "Experiences of the Nurse-Midwife in the Kentucky Mountains." *Nation's Health* 8, no. 12 (December 1926): 2–5.

Callahan, James Morton. *History of West Virginia Old and New, with West Virginia Biography*. 3 vols. Chicago: American Historical Society, 1923.

Campbell, John C. *The Southern Highlander and His Homeland*. 1921. Reprint, Lexington: University Press of Kentucky, 1969.

Eller, C. Howe. "Rural Health Service in Virginia." *University of Virginia Newsletter* 8, no. 15 (May 1937): 1–3.

Ely, William. *The Big Sandy: A History of the People and Country from Earliest Settlement to the Present Time*. 1887. Reprint, Baltimore: Genealogical Publishing Company, 1969.

Farm Foundation. *Medical Care and Health Services for Rural People: A Study Prepared as a Result of a Conference Held at Chicago, Illinois, April 11–13, 1944, Sponsored by the Farm Foundation*. Chicago: Farm Foundation, 1944.

Flexner, Abraham. *Medical Education in the United States and Canada: A Report to the Carnegie Foundation for the Advancement of Teaching*. 1910. Reprint, New York: Arno Press, 1972.

Frankel, Lee, and Louis Dublin. *Sickness among Coal Miners and Their Families*. New York: Metropolitan Life Insurance Company, 1917.

Furman, Lucy. *Mothering on Perilous*. New York: Macmillan, 1915.

———. *The Quare Women*. Boston: Atlantic Monthly Press, 1923.

———. *Sight to the Blind*. New York: Macmillan, 1914.

Fuson, Henry Harvey. *History of Bell County*. New York: Hobson, 1947.

Handy, Henry Brantly. *The Social Recorder of Virginia*. Richmond: Social Recorder of Virginia Publishing, 1928.

Harman, John Newton. *Annals of Tazewell County, Virginia, from 1800 to 1924*. Richmond: W. C. Hill, 1925.

Harvey, Vera Andrew. *The Silver Gleam: Pageant and History of the West Virginia Federation of Women's Clubs*. Charleston: Privately published, 1929.

Higginbotham, Phyllis. "From Our Mountain Nurses." *Southern Mountain Life and Work* 1, no. 3 (October 1925): 26–28.

———. "Pages from a Diary." *Southern Mountain Life and Work* 2, no. 3 (October 1926): 28–29.

Hummell, B. L., and C. G. Bennett. *Magnitude of the Emergency Relief Administration in Rural Virginia*. Blacksburg: Virginia Polytechnic Institute, 1937.

Jillson, Williard Rouse. *The Coal Industry in Kentucky*. Frankfort: Kentucky Geological Survey, 1924.

Johnson, Charles. *A Narrative History of Wise County, Virginia*. Norton, Va.: Norton Press, 1938.

Jones, W. H. *Annual Report of the State Department of Mines for the Year Ending December, 1925*. Charleston: News Mail, 1926.

Kaufmann, Maurice. *The Misadventures of an Appalachian Doctor: Mountain Medicine in the 1930s.* N.p.: Privately published, 1982.

Kephart, Horace. *Our Southern Highlanders.* New York: Outing, 1913.

Kirk, John W. *Progressive West Virginians.* Wheeling: Wheeling Intelligencer, 1923.

Lee, Howard B. *Bloodletting in Appalachia: The Story of West Virginia's Four Major Mine Wars and Other Thrilling Incidents of Its Coal Fields.* Parsons, W.Va.: McClain, 1969.

———. *Looking Backwards One Hundred Years in Appalachia.* Parsons, W.Va.: McClain, 1981.

Maury, M. F. *The Resources of the Coal Fields of the Upper Kanawha, with a Sketch of the Iron Belt of Virginia Setting Forth Some of Their Markets and Means of Development.* Baltimore: Sherwood, 1873.

Miles, Emma Bell. *The Spirit of the Mountains.* 1905. Reprint, Knoxville: University of Tennessee Press, 1975.

Polk, R. L. *Polk's Medical and Surgical Directory of the United States.* Detroit: R. L. Polk, 1886.

———. *Polk's Medical and Surgical Register of North America.* Detroit: R. L. Polk, 1896.

———. *Polk's Medical Register of North America.* Detroit: R. L. Polk, 1906.

———. *Polk's Medical Register of the United States and Canada.* Detroit: R. L. Polk, 1917.

———. *R. L. Polk and Company's Bluefield, West Virginia, Directory.* Pittsburgh: R. L. Polk, 1920–33.

Ryburn, Mrs. White M., Ellen S. Bowen, and Mrs. J. W. Walker. *Women of Old Abingdon.* Pulaski, Va.: B. D. Smith, 1937.

Sloop, Mary Martin. *Miracle in the Hills.* New York: McGraw-Hill, 1953.

Stucky, J. A. "Trachoma among the Natives of the Mountains of Eastern Kentucky." *Journal of the American Medical Association* 61 (27 September 1913): 520–21.

Tobey, James. *The Children's Bureau: Its History, Activities, and Organization.* Baltimore: Johns Hopkins University Press, 1925.

Ulrich, Mrs. Herbert. *The Right Side of the Caduceus: The First Fifty Years, 1922–1972.* Chicago: American Medical Association, 1972.

Ulrich, Laurel Thatcher. *A Midwife's Tale: The Life of Martha Ballard, Based on Her Diary.* New York: Vintage, 1990.

Webber, Gustavus A. *The Women's Bureau: Its History, Activities, and Organization.* Baltimore: Johns Hopkins University Press, 1922.

White, Martha E. D. "The Work of the Woman's Club." *Atlantic Monthly* 93, no. 559 (May 1904): 614–23.

Willeford, Mary B. "Income and Health in Remote Rural Areas: A Study of Four Hundred Families in Leslie County, Kentucky." Ph.D. diss., Columbia University, 1933.

Writers' Program of the Works Progress Administration. *Virginia: A Guide to the Old Dominion.* New York: Oxford University Press, 1964.

Government Publications

Annual Report of the State Board of Health and the State Health Commission to the Governor of Virginia for the Fiscal Year Ending September 30, 1919. Richmond: Davis Bottoms, 1920.

Board of Health of the State of Kentucky. *Bulletin of the State Board of Health of Kentucky.* Vols. 1–25. 1911–36.

Board of Health of the State of Virginia. *Report of the State Board of Health and the State Health Commissioner.* 1911–36.

———. *Virginia Health Bulletin.* Vols. 1–28. 1908–36.

Board of Health of the State of West Virginia. *Biennial Report of the Board of Health of the State of West Virginia and Report of Vital and Mortuary Statistics.* 1881–1936.

———. *Quarterly Bulletin of the West Virginia Department of Health.* Vols. 1–32. 1913–35.

Federal Emergency Relief Administration. *Final Report of the Federal Emergency Relief Administration.* Washington, D.C.: GPO, 1937.

Garnett, William Edward, and Allen David Edwards. *Virginia's Marginal Population: A Study in Rural Poverty.* Bulletin 335. Blacksburg: Virginia Agricultural Experiment Station, 1941.

Hunt, Edward, F. G. Tryon, and Joseph H. Willits. *What the Coal Commission Found.* Baltimore: Williams and Wilkins, 1925.

Laing, John. *Annual Report of the Department of Mines for the Year Ending June 30th, 1910.* Charleston: News Mail, 1911.

Logan County Births, 1872–1900, Dingess Family Bible. North Manchester, Ind.: Heckman, n.d.

McGill, Nettie. *The Welfare of Children in the Bituminous Coal Mining Communities in West Virginia.* U.S. Department of Labor, Children's Bureau. Washington, D.C.: GPO, 1923.

Paul, James W. *Nineteenth Annual Report: Coal Mines in the State of West Virginia, U.S.A., for the Year Ending June 30, 1901.* Charleston: Tribune Printers, 1901.

Ransom, Jane. "Bureau of Public Health Nursing." In *Annual Report of the State Board of Health and the State Health Commission to the Governor of Virginia for the Fiscal Year Ending September 30, 1919.* Richmond: Davis Bottoms, 1920.

Roberts, Lydia. *The Nutrition and Care of Children in a Mountain County of Kentucky.* U.S. Department of Labor, Children's Bureau. Washington, D.C.: GPO, 1922.

Trapnell, W. C., and Ralph Ilsey. *The Bituminous Coal Industry, with a Survey of Competing Fuels.* Federal Emergency Relief Administration. Washington, D.C.: GPO, 1935.

U.S. Coal Commission. *Report of the United States Coal Commission, Part III.* Washington, D.C.: GPO, 1923.

U.S. Department of Commerce, Bureau of the Census. *Census of the United States.* Washington, D.C.: GPO, 1880–1920.

U.S. Department of the Interior, Coal Mines Administration. *A Medical Survey of the Bituminous Coal Industry.* Washington, D.C.: GPO, 1947.

U.S. Senate, Committee on Manufacturers. *Hearings before a Subcommittee of the Committee on Manufacturers, United States Senate, Seventy-second Congress, First Session, on Senate Resolution 178, a Resolution for the Investigation of Conditions in the Coal Fields of Harlan and Bell Counties, Kentucky.* 72d Cong., 1st sess., 1932.

Veazey, Oscar. *First Annual Report of the State Inspector of Mines, Issued to the Governor of the State of West Virginia for the Year 1882.* Wheeling: Charles A. Tanney, 1884.

Journals and Yearbooks

Frontier Nursing Service. *Quarterly Bulletin of the Frontier Nursing Service*. Vols. 1–11. 1925–41.

Graduate Nurses' Association of Virginia. *Bits of News from Headquarters, Graduate State Nurses' Association of Virginia*. Vols. 1–4. 1932–36.

Kentucky State Medical Association. *Kentucky Medical Journal*. Vols. 1–34. 1902–36.

Medical Society of Virginia. *Virginia Medical Monthly*. Vols. 1–63. 1873–1936.

Pine Mountain Settlement School. *Notes from the Pine Mountain Settlement School*. Vols. 1–8. 1928–36.

Southern Mountain Life and Work. Vols. 1–11. 1925–36.

Virginia Federation of Women's Clubs. *Bulletin of the Virginia Federation of Women's Clubs*. Vol. 1. 1926.

———. *Club Life in the Old Dominion*. Vols. 1–2. 1922–23.

———. *Virginia Federation of Women's Clubs Yearbook*. 1911–12, 1923–24, 1924–25, 1929–30.

Virginia Medical Society. *Virginia Medical Monthly*. 1890–1930.

West Virginia Federation of Women's Clubs. *West Virginia Clubwoman*. 1917–24.

———. *West Virginia Federation of Women's Clubs Manual*. 1908–11.

———. *West Virginia Federation of Women's Clubs Yearbook*. 1904–36.

West Virginia State Medical Association. *Transactions of the Medical Society of the State of West Virginia, Instituted April 10, 1867, Together with the Code of Ethics and Bylaws*. Wheeling: Frew, Hagans, and Hall, 1868.

———. *West Virginia Medical Journal*. Vols. 1–36. 1904–40.

West Virginia State Nurses' Association. *Weather Vane*. Vols. 2–9. 1927–36.

Newspapers

Bluefield Daily Telegraph
Charleston Gazette
Louisville Courier Journal
New Dominion
Staunton News Leader
Williamson Daily News

Secondary Sources

Abramovitz, Mimi. *Regulating the Lives of Women: Social Welfare Policy from Colonial Times to the Present*. Boston: South End Press, 1988.

Andrew Donnally Chapter of the Daughters of the American Revolution. *McDowell County History*. Fort Worth: University Supply and Equipment Company, 1959.

Anglin, Mary. "Activists and Advocates as Actors in Health Care." In *Sowing Seeds in the Mountains: Community-Based Coalitions for Cancer Prevention and Control*, edited by Richard Couto, Nancy Simpson, and Gale Harris, 179–93. Washington,

D.C.: Appalachian Leadership Initiative on Cancer, Cancer Control Sciences Program, Division of Cancer Prevention and Control, National Cancer Institute, 1994.

——. "Lives on the Margin: Rediscovering the Women of Antebellum North Carolina." In *Appalachia in the Making: The Mountain South in the Nineteenth Century*, edited by Mary Beth Pudup, Dwight Billings, and Altina Waller, 185–209. Chapel Hill: University of North Carolina Press, 1995.

——. "A Question of Loyalty: National and Regional Identity in Narratives of Appalachia." *Anthropological Quarterly* 65 (July 1992): 105–16.

Apple, Rima. *Mothers and Medicine: A Social History of Infant Feeding*. Madison: University of Wisconsin Press, 1987.

Armeny, Susan. "Organized Nurses, Women Philanthropists, and the Intellectual Bases for Cooperation among Women." In *Nursing History: New Perspectives, New Possibilities*, edited by Ellen Condliffe Lagemann, 13–46. New York: Teachers' College, Columbia University Press, 1983.

Arnow, Harriet Simpson. *The Dollmaker*. Lexington: University Press of Kentucky, 1954.

Bailey, Benny Ray. "A Case Study of the First Year of the Development of East Kentucky Health Services Center, Inc." Ph.D. diss., Ohio University, 1975.

Baker, Paula. "The Domestication of Politics: Women and American Political Society, 1780–1920." *American Historical Review* 89 (June 1984): 620–47.

Ball, Bonnie. "Tivis Colley Sutherland: Pioneer Doctor of the Frying Pan." *Historical and Biographical Sketches*. Wise, Va.: Clinch Valley College Printing Office, 1972.

Banks, Alan. "Class Formation in the Southeastern Kentucky Coalfields." In *Appalachia in the Making: The Mountain South in the Nineteenth Century*, edited by Mary Beth Pudup, Dwight Billings, and Altina Waller, 321–46. Chapel Hill: University of North Carolina Press, 1995.

Barney, Sandra. "Health Services in a Stranded Community: Scotts Run, 1920–1947." *West Virginia History* 53 (1994): 42–59.

Batteau, Allen, ed. *Appalachia and America: Autonomy and Regional Dependence*. Lexington: University Press of Kentucky, 1983.

——. *The Invention of Appalachia*. Tucson: University of Arizona Press, 1990.

Beardsley, Edward. *A History of Neglect: Health Care for Blacks and Mill Workers in the Twentieth Century South*. Knoxville: University of Tennessee Press, 1987.

Beaver, Patricia D. "Symbols and Social Organization in an Appalachian Mountain Community." Ph.D. diss., Duke University, 1976.

Becker, Dorothy. "Exit Lady Bountiful: The Volunteer and the Professional Social Worker." *Social Service Review* 34 (March 1964): 57–72.

Becker, Jane. *Selling Tradition: Appalachia and the Construction of an American Folk, 1930–1940*. Chapel Hill: University of North Carolina Press, 1998.

Becker, Martha Jane Williams. *Bramwell: The Diary of a Millionaire Coal Town*. Chapmanville, W.Va.: The Printers, 1988.

Behringer, Bruce. "Health Care Services in Appalachia." In *Sowing Seeds in the Mountains: Community-Based Coalitions for Cancer Prevention and Control*, edited by Richard Couto, Nancy Simpson, and Gale Harris, 62–80. Washington,

D.C.: Appalachian Leadership Initiative on Cancer, Cancer Control Sciences Program, Division of Cancer Prevention and Control, National Cancer Institute, 1994.

Belanger, Ruth. "Midwives' Tales." *Goldenseal* 5 (October–December 1979): 42–46.

Bender, Thomas. *Community and Social Change in America*. New Brunswick: Rutgers University Press, 1978.

Berlant, Jeffrey Lionel. *Profession and Monopoly: A Study of Medicine in the United States and Great Britain*. Berkeley: University of California Press, 1975.

Bickley, Ancella. "Midwifery in West Virginia." *West Virginia History* 49 (1990): 55–67.

Billings, Dwight, Mary Beth Pudup, and Altina Waller. "Taking Exception with Exceptionalism: The Emergence and Transformation of Historical Studies of Appalachia." In *Appalachia in the Making: The Mountain South in the Nineteenth Century*, edited by Mary Beth Pudup, Dwight Billings, and Altina Waller, 1–24. Chapel Hill: University of North Carolina Press, 1995.

Blair, Karen. *The Clubwoman as Feminist: True Womanhood Redefined, 1868–1914*. New York: Gardner, 1980.

Bledstein, Burton J. *The Culture of Professionalism: The Middle Class and the Development of Higher Education in America*. New York: Norton, 1976.

Blee, Kathleen, and Dwight Billings. "Family Strategies in a Subsistence Economy: Beech Creek, Kentucky, 1850–1942." *Sociological Perspectives* 33, no. 1 (1990): 63–88.

Blumer, Herbert. *Industrialization as an Agent of Social Change*. New York: Aldine de Gruyter, 1990.

Bonner, Thomas. *Becoming a Physician: Medical Education in Britain, France, Germany, and the United States*. Cambridge: Harvard University Press, 1995.

Bordin, Ruth. *Women and Temperance: The Quest for Power and Liberty, 1873–1900*. New Brunswick: Rutgers University Press, 1990.

Borst, Charlotte. *Catching Babies: The Professionalization of Childbirth, 1870–1920*. Cambridge: Harvard University Press, 1995.

———. "Wisconsin's Midwives as Working Women: Immigrant Midwives and the Limits of a Traditional Occupation, 1870–1920." *Journal of American Ethnic History* 8, no. 2 (Spring 1989): 24–50.

Boston Women's Health Book Collective. *Our Bodies, Ourselves: Updated and Expanded for the '90s*. New York: Simon and Schuster, 1992.

Brickman, Jane Pacht. "Public Health, Midwives, and Nurses, 1880–1930." In *Nursing History: New Perspectives, New Possibilities*, edited by Ellen Condliffe Lagemann, 65–88. New York: Teachers' College, Columbia University Press, 1983.

Brown, E. Richard. *Rockefeller Medicine Men: Medicine and Capitalism in America*. Berkeley: University of California Press, 1979.

Buhler-Wilkerson, Karen. *False Dawn: The Rise and Decline of Public Health Nursing*. New York: Garland, 1989.

Bulmer, Martin, Kevin Bates, and Kathryn Kish Sklar, eds. *The Social Survey in*

Historical Perspective, 1880–1940. Cambridge: Cambridge University Press, 1991.

Burrow, James G. *AMA: Voice of American Medicine.* Baltimore: Johns Hopkins University Press, 1963.

———. *Organized Medicine in the Progressive Era: The Move toward Monopoly.* Baltimore: Johns Hopkins University Press, 1977.

Carson, Mina. *Settlement Folk: Social Thought and the American Settlement Movement, 1885–1930.* Chicago: University of Chicago Press, 1990.

Cassedy, James. "Why Self-Help?: Americans Alone with Their Disease, 1800–1850." In *Medicine without Doctors: Home Health Care in American History,* edited by Guenter B. Risse, Ronald Numbers, and Judith Walzer Leavitt, 31–48. New York: Science History Publication, 1977.

Chambers, Clarke. *Seedtime of Reform: American Social Service and Social Action, 1918–1933.* Westport, Conn.: Greenwood Press, 1980.

———. "Toward a Redefinition of Welfare History." *Journal of American History* 73 (September 1986): 407–33.

Cirillo, Marie. "Every Mountain Hollow." In *Women Activists: Challenging the Abuse of Power,* edited by Anne Witte Garland, 3–16. New York: Feminist Press, 1988.

Comstock, Jim. *West Virginia Women.* Richwood, W.Va.: Privately published, 1974.

Corbin, David Alan. *Life, Work, and Rebellion in the Coal Fields: The Southern West Virginia Miners, 1880–1922.* Urbana: University of Illinois Press, 1981.

Cornett, Judy Gail. "Angel for the Blind: The Public Triumphs and Private Tragedy of Linda Neville." Ph.D. diss., University of Kentucky, 1993.

Cott, Nancy. *The Grounding of Modern Feminism.* New Haven: Yale University Press, 1987.

———. "What's in a Name?: The Limits of 'Social Feminism,' or Expanding the Vocabulary of Women's History." *Journal of American History* 76 (December 1989): 809–29.

Couto, Richard. *An American Challenge: A Report on Economic Trends and Social Issues in Appalachia.* Dubuque: Kendall/Hunt, 1994.

———. "Appalachian Health Innovations." In *American Issues in Appalachia,* edited by Alan Batteau, 168–88. Lexington: University Press of Kentucky, 1983.

———. "The Political Economy of Appalachian Health." In *Health in Appalachia: Proceedings of the 1988 University of Kentucky Conference on Appalachia,* 5–16. Lexington: University Press of Kentucky, 1989.

———. "Poverty, Politics, and Health Care: The Experience of One Appalachian County." Ph.D. diss., University of Kentucky, 1974.

———. *Poverty, Politics, and Health Care: An Appalachian Experience.* New York: Praeger, 1975.

Couto, Richard, Nancy Simpson, and Gale Harris, eds. *Sowing Seeds in the Mountains: Community-Based Coalitions for Cancer Prevention and Control.* Washington, D.C.: Appalachian Leadership Initiative on Cancer, Cancer Control Sciences Program, Division of Cancer Prevention and Control, National Cancer Institute, 1994.

Cox, William E. "McKendree No. 2: The Story of West Virginia's Miners Hospitals." *Goldenseal* 7 (Fall 1981): 36–40.

Crellin, John K., and Jane Philpott. *Trying to Give Ease.* Vol. 1 of *Herbal Medicine Past and Present.* Durham: Duke University Press, 1990.

Crocker, Ruth Hutchinson. *Social Work and Social Order: The Settlement Movement in Two Industrial Cities, 1889–1930.* Urbana: University of Illinois Press, 1992.

Cumbler, John T. "The Politics of Charity: Gender and Class in Late Nineteenth Century Charity Policy." *Journal of Social History* 14 (Fall 1980): 99–111.

Dammann, Nancy. *A Social History of the Frontier Nursing Service.* Sun City, Ariz.: Social Change Press, 1982.

Davis, Allen F. *Spearheads for Reform: The Social Settlements and the Progressive Movement, 1890–1914.* New Brunswick: Rutgers University Press, 1984.

DeClerq, Eugene, and Richard Lacroix. "The Immigrant Midwives of Lawrence: The Conflict between Law and Culture." *Bulletin of the History of Medicine* 59, no. 2 (1985): 232–46.

Donegan, Jane. *Women and Men Midwives: Medicine, Morality, and Misogyny in Early America.* Westport, Conn.: Greenwood Press, 1978.

Douglas, Mary. *How Institutions Think.* Syracuse: Syracuse University Press, 1986.

Doyal, Lesley, and Imogene Pennell. *The Political Economy of Health.* Boston: South End Press, 1981.

——. *What Makes Women Sick: Gender and the Political Economy of Health.* New Brunswick: Rutgers University Press, 1995.

Duffy, John. "The American Medical Profession and Public Health: From Support to Ambivalence." *Bulletin of the History of Medicine* 53 (Spring 1979): 1–22.

——. *The Sanitarians: A History of American Public Health.* Urbana: University of Illinois Press, 1990.

Dunaway, Wilma A. *The First American Frontier: Transition to Capitalism in Southern Appalachia, 1700–1860.* Chapel Hill: University of North Carolina Press, 1996.

Dye, Nancy Schrom. "Mary Breckinridge, the Frontier Nursing Service, and the Introduction of Nurse-Midwifery in the United States." *Bulletin of the History of Medicine* 57 (Winter 1983): 485–507.

Effland, Anne Wallace. "The Woman Suffrage Movement in West Virginia, 1867–1920." Master's thesis, West Virginia University, 1983.

Efird, Cathy Melvin. "A Geography of Lay Midwifery in Appalachian North Carolina, 1925–1950." Ph.D. diss., University of North Carolina, 1985.

Ehrenreich, Barbara, and Deidre English. *Complaints and Disorders: The Sexual Politics of Sickness.* New York: Feminist Press, 1973.

——. *For Her Own Good: One Hundred and Fifty Years of the Experts' Advice to Women.* New York: Doubleday, 1978.

Ehrenreich, John H. *The Altruistic Imagination: A History of Social Work and Social Policy in the United States.* Ithaca: Cornell University Press, 1985.

Eisenstadt, S. N. *Tradition, Change, and Modernity.* New York: John Wiley and Sons, 1973.

Elkins, Eugene, and Larry Young. *Public Health Administration in West Virginia.*

Morgantown: West Virginia University Bureau for Government Research, 1956.

Eller, Ronald. *Miners, Millhands, and Mountaineers: Industrialization of the Appalachian South, 1880–1930.* Knoxville: University of Tennessee Press, 1982.

Ellis, John H. *Medicine in Kentucky.* Lexington: University Press of Kentucky, 1977.

Evans, Sara M., and Harry C. Boyte. *Free Spaces: The Sources of Democratic Change in America.* New York: Harper and Row, 1986.

Fass, Paula. *The Damned and the Beautiful: American Youth in the 1920s.* New York: Oxford University Press, 1977.

Fishbein, Morris. *History of the American Medical Association.* Philadelphia: W. B. Saunders, 1947.

Flanagan, Maureen A. "Gender and Urban Political Reform: The City Club and the Woman's City Club of Chicago in the Progressive Era." *American Historical Review* 95 (October 1990): 1032–50.

Flora, Cornelia B., and Jan L. Flora. "Entrepreneurial Social Infrastructure: A Necessary Ingredient." *Annals of the American Academy of Political and Social Science* 529 (September 1993): 48–58.

Forderhase, Nancy K. " 'The Clear Call of Thoroughbred Women': The Kentucky Federation of Women's Clubs and the Crusade for Educational Reform." *Register of the Kentucky Historical Society* 83, no. 1 (Winter 1985): 19–35.

———. "Eve Returns to the Garden: Women Reformers in Appalachian Kentucky in the Early Twentieth Century." *Register of the Kentucky Historical Society* 85, no. 3 (1987): 237–61.

Foucault, Michel. *Discipline and Punish: The Birth of the Prison.* Translated by Alan Sheridan. New York: Random House, 1991.

———. *Power / Knowledge: Selected Interviews and Other Writings, 1972–1977.* Edited by Colin Gordon; translated by Colin Gordon, Leo Marshall, John Mepham, and Kate Soper. New York: Pantheon Books, 1977.

Frankel, Noralee, and Nancy S. Dye, eds. *Gender, Class, Race, and Reform in the Progressive Era.* Lexington: University Press of Kentucky, 1991.

Frazier, Claude, and F. K. Brown. *Miners and Medicine: West Virginia Memories.* Norman: University of Oklahoma Press, 1992.

Friedson, Eliot. "Are the Professions Necessary?" In *The Authority of Experts,* edited by Thomas Haskell. Bloomington: Indiana University Press, 1984.

———. *Professional Dominance: The Social Structure of Medical Care.* New York: Atherton, 1970.

———. *Profession of Medicine.* New York: Dodd and Mead, 1970.

———. "Professions in Contemporary Society." *American Behavioral Scientist* 14 (1971): 37–54.

Funk, Fanchon Felice. "Health Attitudes and Practices in an Isolated Appalachian Valley." Ed.D. thesis, University of Tennessee, 1970.

Gaventa, John. *Power and Powerlessness: Quiescence and Rebellion in an Appalachian Valley.* Urbana: University of Illinois Press, 1980.

Gevitz, Norman. *The D.O.'s: Osteopathic Medicine in America.* Baltimore: Johns Hopkins University Press, 1982.

Ginzberg, Lori. *Women and the Work of Benevolence: Morality, Politics, and Class in the Nineteenth Century.* New Haven: Yale University Press, 1990.

Girling, John. *Capital and Power: Political Economy and Social Transformation.* London: Croom Helm, 1987.

Gordon, Linda. "Black and White Visions of Welfare: Women's Welfare Activism, 1890–1945." *Journal of American History* 78 (September 1991): 559–90.

———. *Heroes of Their Own Lives: The Politics and History of Family Violence, Boston, 1880–1960.* New York: Viking, 1988.

Gramsci, Antonio. *Selections from the Prison Notebooks.* Edited and translated by Q. Hoare and G. N. Smith. New York: International Publishers, 1971.

Graves, Glenna Horne. "In the Morning We Had Bulldog Gravy: Women in the Coal Camps of the Appalachian South, 1900–1940." Ph.D. diss., University of Kentucky, 1993.

Grew, Raymond. "Modernization and Its Discontents." *American Behavioral Scientist* 21 (November–December 1977): 289–312.

Hahn, Steven. *The Roots of Southern Populism: Yeoman Farmers and the Transformation of the Georgia Upcountry, 1850–1890.* New York: Oxford University Press, 1982.

Hahn, Steven, and Jonathan Prude, eds. *The Countryside in the Age of Capitalist Transformation.* Chapel Hill: University of North Carolina Press, 1985.

Hay, Melba Porter. "Madeline McDowell Breckinridge: Kentucky Suffragist and Progressive Reformer." Ph.D. diss., University of Kentucky, 1980.

Hefner, Loretta. "The National Women's Relief Society and the U.S. Sheppard-Towner Act." *Utah Historical Quarterly* 50, no. 3 (Summer 1982): 254–67.

Heinemann, Ronald. *Depression and New Deal in Virginia: The Enduring Dominion.* Charlottesville: University of Virginia Press, 1983.

Hennen, John C. *The Americanization of West Virginia: Creating a Modern Industrial State, 1916–1925.* Lexington: University Press of Kentucky, 1996.

Herrin, Dean. "Breaking the Stillness: The Coal Industry and the Transformation of Appalachian Virginia, 1880–1920." Ph.D. diss., University of Delaware, 1991.

Hewitt, Nancy. *Women's Activism and Social Change: Rochester, New York, 1822–1872.* Ithaca: Cornell University Press, 1984.

Hibbard, Walter. *Virginia Coal: An Abridged History and Complete Data Manual of Virginia Coal Production/Consumption from 1748–1988.* Blacksburg: Virginia Center for Coal and Energy Research, Virginia Polytechnic Institute and State University, 1990.

Hill, Patricia Evridge. "Go Tell It on the Mountain: Hilla Sheriff and Public Health in the South Carolina Piedmont, 1929 to 1940." *American Journal of Public Health* 85, no. 4 (1995): 578–84.

Hiott, Susan Giaimo. "Osteopathy in South Carolina: The Struggle for Recognition." *South Carolina Historical Magazine* 91, no. 3 (July 1990): 184–97.

Hiscoe, Helen B. *Appalachian Passage.* Athens: University of Georgia Press, 1991.

Hoffert, Sylvia. *Private Matters: American Attitudes toward Childbearing and Infant Nurture in the Urban North, 1800–1860.* Urbana: University of Illinois Press, 1989.

Hoffman, Lily M. *The Politics of Knowledge: Activist Movements in Medicine and Planning.* Albany: State University of New York Press, 1989.

Hofstadter, Richard. *The Age of Reform: From Bryan to F.D.R.* New York: Vintage, 1955.

Hogshead, Norma. *Past Presidents of the Woman's Auxiliary to the West Virginia State Medical Association.* Parkersburg, W.Va.: McGlothin, 1949.

Hopp, Joyce W. *Babies in Her Saddlebags: Adventures of a Kentucky Midwife.* Boise, Idaho: Pacific Press Publishing Association, 1986.

Howell, Colin D. "Medical Professionalization and the Social Transformation of the Maritimes, 1850–1950." *Journal of Canadian Studies* 27, no. 1 (Spring 1992): 5–20.

Huff, Marlene. "The Effects of the UMWA upon the Reform of the Company Doctor System." Paper presented at the Appalachian Studies Conference, 1993; copy in author's possession.

Illich, Ivan. *Medical Nemesis: The Expropriation of Health.* London: Calder and Boyars, 1975.

Inscoe, John. *Mountain Masters, Slavery, and the Sectional Crisis in Western North Carolina.* Knoxville: University of Tennessee Press, 1989.

Karger, Howard Jacob. *The Sentinels of Order: A Study of Social Control and the Minneapolis Settlement House Movement, 1915–1950.* Lanham, Md.: University Press of America, 1987.

Kaufert, Patricia A., and John D. O'Neil. "Cooptation and Control: The Reconstruction of Inuit Birth." *Medical Anthropology Quarterly* 4 (December 1990): 427–42.

Kaufman, Martin. *Homeopathy in America: The Rise and Fall of a Medical Heresy.* Baltimore: Johns Hopkins University Press, 1971.

Kegley, Mary B. *Wythe County, Virginia: A Bicentennial History.* Marceline, Mo.: Walsworth, 1989.

Keith, Jeanette. *Country People in the New South: Tennessee's Upper Cumberland.* Chapel Hill: University of North Carolina Press, 1996.

Kerber, Linda, Alice Kessler-Harris, and Kathryn Kish Sklar, eds. *American History as Women's History: New Feminist Essays.* Chapel Hill: University of North Carolina Press, 1995.

Kett, Joseph. *Formation of the American Medical Profession.* New Haven: Yale University Press, 1968.

Kirschner, Don S. *The Paradox of Professionalism: Reform and Public Service in Urban America, 1900–1940.* Westport, Conn.: Greenwood Press, 1986.

Kobrin, Frances E. "The American Midwife Controversy: A Crisis of Professionalization." *Bulletin of the History of Medicine* 40, no. 4 (1966): 350–63.

Koven, Seth, and Sonya Michel. *Mothers of a New World: Maternalist Politics and the Origins of Welfare States.* New York: Routledge, 1993.

———. "Womanly Duties: Maternalist Politics and the Origins of Welfare States

in France, Germany, Great Britain, and the United States, 1880–1920."
American Historical Review 95, no. 4 (October 1990): 1076–1108.

Kulikoff, Allan. "The Transformation to Capitalism in Rural America." *William and Mary Quarterly* 46 (January 1989): 120–44.

Kunzel, Regina. *Fallen Women, Problem Girls: Unmarried Mothers and the Professionalization of Social Work, 1890–1945.* New Haven: Yale University Press, 1993.

Ladd-Taylor, Molly. " 'Grannies' and 'Spinsters': Midwife Education under the Sheppard-Towner Act." *Journal of Social History* 22 (Winter 1988): 255–75.

———. *Mother-Work: Women, Child Welfare, and the State, 1890–1930.* Urbana: University of Illinois Press, 1994.

———. *Raising a Baby the Government Way: Mothers' Letters to the Children's Bureau.* New Brunswick: Rutgers University Press, 1986.

———. "Toward Defining Maternalism in U.S. History." *Journal of Women's History* 5, no. 2 (Fall 1993): 109–26.

Ladd-Taylor, Molly, and Laurie Umansky. *"Bad" Mothers: The Politics of Blame in Twentieth Century America.* New York: New York University Press, 1998.

Larson, Magali Sarfatti. "The Production of Expertise and the Constitution of Expert Power." In *The Authority of Experts,* edited by Thomas Haskell, 28–83. Bloomington: Indiana University Press, 1984.

———. *The Rise of Professionalism: A Sociological Analysis.* Berkeley: University of California Press, 1977.

Lasch-Quinn, Elizabeth. *Black Neighbors: Race and the Limits of Reform in the American Settlement House Movement, 1890–1945.* Chapel Hill: University of North Carolina Press, 1993.

Leavitt, Judith Walzer. *Brought to Bed: Childbearing in America, 1750–1950.* New York: Oxford University Press, 1986.

———. "Gendered Expectations: Women and Early Twentieth Century Public Health." In *U.S. History as Women's History: New Feminist Essays,* edited by Linda K. Kerber, Alice Kessler-Harris, and Kathryn Kish Sklar. Chapel Hill: University of North Carolina Press, 1995.

———. *The Healthiest City: Milwaukee and the Politics of Health Reform.* Princeton: Princeton University Press, 1982.

———. " 'Science' Enters the Birthing Room: Obstetrics in America since the Eighteenth Century." *Journal of American History* 70, no. 2 (1983): 281–304.

———. *Typhoid Mary: Captive to the Public's Health.* Boston: Beacon Press, 1996.

———. " 'Typhoid Mary' Strikes Back: Bacteriological Theory and Practice in Early Twentieth-Century Public Health." *Isis* 83, no. 4 (December 1992): 608–29.

———. " 'A Worrying Profession': The Domestic Environment of Medical Practice in Mid-Nineteenth Century America." *Bulletin of the History of Medicine* 69, no. 1 (1995): 1–29.

Leavitt, Judith Walzer, and Ronald L. Numbers, eds. *Sickness and Health in America: Readings in the History of Medicine and Public Health.* Madison: University of Wisconsin Press, 1985.

Lebsock, Suzanne. *Free Women of Petersburg: Status and Culture in a Southern Town, 1784–1860.* New York: Norton, 1985.

———. *Virginia Women, 1600–1945: "A Share of Honour."* Richmond: Virginia State Library, 1987.

———. "Woman Suffrage and White Supremacy: A Virginia Case Study." In *Visible Women: New Essays in American Activism*, edited by Nancy Hewitt and Suzanne Lebsock, 62–100. Urbana: University of Illinois Press, 1993.

Lemon, Stanley J. *The Woman Citizen: Social Feminism in the 1920s.* Urbana: University of Illinois Press, 1973.

Lewis, Ronald L. "Appalachian Restructuring in Historical Perspective: Coal, Culture, and Social Change in West Virginia." Research paper no. 9102. Morgantown, W.Va.: Regional Research Institute, 1992.

———. "Railroads, Deforestation, and the Transformation of Agriculture in the West Virginia Back Counties, 1880–1920." In *Appalachia in the Making: The Mountain South in the Nineteenth Century*, edited by Mary Beth Pudup, Dwight Billings, and Altina Waller, 297–320. Chapel Hill: University of North Carolina Press, 1995.

———. *Transforming the Appalachian Countryside: Railroads, Deforestation, and Social Change in West Virginia, 1880–1929.* Chapel Hill: University of North Carolina Press, 1998.

Lieberman, Jethro K. *The Tyranny of the Experts: How Professionals Are Closing the Open Society.* New York: Walker, 1970.

Link, William A. "Privies, Progressivism, and Public Schools: Health Reform and Education in the Rural South, 1909–1920." *Journal of Southern History* 54, no. 4 (November 1988): 623–42.

Lissak, Rivka Shpak. *Pluralism and Progressives: Hull House and the New Immigrants, 1890–1919.* Chicago: University of Chicago Press, 1989.

Litoff, Judith Barrett. *American Midwives, 1860 to the Present.* Westport, Conn.: Greenwood Press, 1978.

Logan, Onnie Lee. *Motherwit: An Alabama Midwife's Tale.* Edited by Katherine Clark. New York: Dutton, 1989.

Lopes, Daniel, Joan Moser, and Annie Louise Perkinson. *Appalachian Folk Medicine: Native Plants and Healing Traditions.* Swannanoa, N.C.: Warren Wilson Press, 1997.

Lubove, Roy. *Professionalism and Altruism: The Emergence of Social Work as a Career, 1880–1930.* New York: Atheneum, 1980.

Ludmerer, Kenneth. *Learning to Heal: The Development of American Medical Education.* New York: Basic Books, 1985.

McCarthy, Kathleen D., ed. *Lady Bountiful Revisited: Women, Philanthropy, and Power.* New Brunswick: Rutgers University Press, 1990.

McGehee, Stuart. "Sawbones: The Company Doctor Gets His Due." *Coal People Magazine*, August 1990, 11–15.

McMillen, Sally. *Motherhood in the Old South: Pregnancy, Childbirth, and Infant Rearing.* Baton Rouge: Louisiana State University Press, 1990.

Maggard, Sally Ward. "Class and Gender: New Theoretical Priorities in Appalachian Studies." In *The Impact of Institutions in Appalachia: Proceedings of the Eighth Annual Appalachian Studies Conference*, edited by James Lloyd and Ann Campbell, 100–113. Boone, N.C.: Appalachian Consortium Press, 1986.

———. "From Farmers to Miners: The Decline of Agriculture in Eastern Kentucky." In *Science and Agricultural Development*, edited by Lawrence Bush, 25–66. Totowa, N.J.: Allanheld, Osmun, 1981.

———. "From the Farm to the Coal Camp to the Back Office to McDonald's: Living in the Midst of Appalachia's Latest Transformation." *Journal of the Appalachian Studies Association* 6 (1994): 14–38.

———. "Gender, Race, and Place: Confounding Labor Activism in Appalachia." In *Neither Separate Nor Equal: Women, Race, and Class in the U.S. South*, edited by Barbara Ellen Smith, 185–206. Philadelphia: Temple University Press, 1999.

Markowitz, Gerald, and David Rosner. "Doctors in Crisis: Medical Education and Medical Reform during the Progressive Era, 1895–1915." In *Health Care in America: Essays in Social History*, edited by Susan Reverby and David Rosner, 185–205. Philadelphia: Temple University Press, 1979.

Maulitz, Russell. " 'Physician versus Bacteriologist': The Ideology of Science in Clinical Medicine." In *The Therapeutic Revolution: Essays in the Social History of American Medicine*, edited by Charles Rosenberg and Morris Vogel, 91–108. Philadelphia: University of Pennsylvania Press, 1979.

Meckel, Richard. *Save the Babies: American Public Health Reform and the Prevention of Infant Mortality*. Baltimore: Johns Hopkins University Press, 1990.

Melosh, Barbara. *"The Physician's Hand": Work Culture and Conflict in American Nursing*. Philadelphia: Temple University Press, 1982.

Mercer County Historical Society. *Mercer County History*. Marceline, Mo.: Walsworth, 1985.

Midgette, Nancy Smith. "In Search of Scientific Legitimacy: Southern Scientists, 1883–1940." *Journal of Southern History* 54, no. 4 (November 1988): 597–622.

———. *To Foster the Spirit of Professionalism*. Tuscaloosa: University of Alabama Press, 1991.

Mulcahy, Richard. "Health Care in the Coal Fields: The Miners Memorial Hospital Association." *Historian* 55, no. 4 (Summer 1993): 641–56.

———. "A New Deal for the Coal Miners: The U.M.W.A. Welfare and Retirement Fund and the Reorganization of Health Care in Appalachia." Paper presented at the Appalachian Studies Conference, 1995; copy in author's possession.

Muncy, Robyn. *Creating a Female Dominion in American Reform, 1890–1935*. New York: Oxford University Press, 1991.

Nash, June, and Max Kirsch. "The Discourse of Medical Science in the Construction of Consensus between Corporation and Community." *Medical Anthropology Quarterly* 2 (June 1988): 158–71.

Navarro, Vicente. *Medicine under Capitalism*. New York: Prodist, 1976.

———. *The Politics of Health Policy: The U.S. Reforms, 1980–1994*. Cambridge: Blackwell, 1994.

Noe, Kenneth. *Southwest Virginia's Railroads: Modernization and the Sectional Crisis*. Urbana: University of Illinois Press, 1994.

Nolan, Robert, and Jerome L. Schwartz, eds. *Rural and Appalachian Health.* Springfield, Ill.: Charles C. Thomas, 1973.

Northington, Etta Belle Walker. *A History of the Virginia Federation of Women's Clubs, 1907–1957.* Richmond: Whittet & Shepperson, 1958.

Norwood, William Frederick. *Medical Education in the United States before the Civil War.* 1944. Reprint, New York: Arno Press and the New York Times, 1971.

Numbers, R. L. *Almost Persuaded: American Physicians and Compulsory Health Insurance, 1912–1920.* Baltimore: Johns Hopkins University Press, 1978.

———. "The Rise and Fall of the American Medical Association." In *Sickness and Health in America: Readings in the History of Medicine and Public Health*, edited by Ronald L. Numbers and Judith Walzer Leavitt, 118–34. Madison: University of Wisconsin Press, 1985.

Odem, Mary. *Delinquent Daughters: Protecting and Policing Adolescent Female Sexuality in the United States, 1885–1920.* Chapel Hill: University of North Carolina Press, 1995.

Osterud, Nancy. *Bonds of Community: The Lives of Farm Women in Nineteenth Century New York.* Ithaca: Cornell University Press, 1991.

Pearce, John Ed. *Days of Darkness: The Feuds of Eastern Kentucky.* Lexington: University Press of Kentucky, 1994.

Peddle, Dorothy Hall. "To Do What's Right." *Southern Exposure* 11 (March–April 1983): 39–43.

Pelligrino, Edmund. "Sociocultural Impact of Modern Therapeutics." In *The Therapeutic Revolution: Essays in the Social History of American Medicine*, edited by Charles Rosenberg and Morris Vogel, 245–66. Philadelphia: University of Pennsylvania Press, 1979.

Petry, Howard. *A Century of Medicine, 1848–1948: The History of the Medical Society of the State of Pennsylvania.* Harrisburg: Medical Society of the State of Pennsylvania, 1952.

Piven, Frances Fox, and Richard A. Cloward. *Poor People's Movements: Why They Succeed, How They Fail.* New York: Vintage, 1977.

———. *Regulating the Poor: The Functions of Public Welfare.* New York: Vintage, 1971.

Ploss, Janet. "A History of the Medical Care Program of the United Mine Workers of America Welfare and Retirement Fund." Master's thesis, Johns Hopkins University, 1981.

Porter, Roy, ed. *The Cambridge Illustrated History of Medicine.* Cambridge: Cambridge University Press, 1996.

Prude, Jonathan. *The Coming of the Industrial Order: Town and Factory in Rural Massachusetts, 1810–1860.* Cambridge: Cambridge University Press, 1983.

Pudup, Mary Beth. "The Boundaries of Class in Preindustrial Appalachia." *Journal of Historical Geography* 15, no. 2 (1989): 139–62.

———. "Land before Coal: Class and Regional Development in Southeast Kentucky." Ph.D. diss., University of California, 1987.

———. "The Limits of Subsistence: Agriculture and Industry in Central Appalachia." *Agricultural History* 64 (1990): 61–89.

———. "Town and Country in the Transformation of Appalachian Kentucky." In

Appalachia in the Making: The Mountain South in the Nineteenth Century, edited by Dwight Billings, Mary Beth Pudup, and Altina Waller, 270–96. Chapel Hill: University of North Carolina Press, 1995.

Pudup, Mary Beth, Dwight Billings, and Altina Waller, eds. *Appalachia in the Making: The Mountain South in the Nineteenth Century*. Chapel Hill: University of North Carolina Press, 1995.

Rakes, Paul. "West Virginia's Entrepreneurial Alliance and the Protection of Business-as-Usual." Unpublished paper in author's possession.

Rayack, Elton. *Professional Power and American Medicine: The Economics of the American Medical Association*. Cleveland: World, 1967.

Reid, Mary Margaret. *Thirty-five Years of the West Virginia State Nurses' Association: A History of Nursing in West Virginia*. Charleston: West Virginia State Nurses' Association, 1942.

Reisman, David. *The Political Economy of Health Care*. New York: St. Martin's, 1993.

Reverby, Susan M. *Ordered to Care: The Dilemma of American Nursing, 1850–1945*. Cambridge: Cambridge University Press, 1987.

Risse, Gunter B., Ronald L. Numbers, and Judith Walzer Leavitt, eds. *Medicine without Doctors: Home Health Care in American History*. New York: Science History Publications, 1977.

Ritchie, Susan. "A Comparison of Infant Mortality in Logan County, West Virginia, in 1872 and 1910." Unpublished paper in the possession of Ronald L. Lewis.

Roberts, Leonard. *Up Cutshin and Down Greasy: Folkways of a Kentucky Family*. Lexington: University Press of Kentucky, 1959.

Rose, Elizabeth. "Taking on a Mother's Job: Day Care in the 1920s and 1930s." In *"Bad" Mothers: The Politics of Blame in Twentieth Century America*, edited by Molly Ladd-Taylor and Laurie Umansky, 67–98. New York: New York University Press, 1998.

Rosen, George. *A History of Public Health*. Baltimore: Johns Hopkins University Press, 1993.

——. *The Structure of American Medical Practice, 1875–1941*. Philadelphia: University of Pennsylvania Press, 1983.

Rosenberg, Charles. *The Care of Strangers: The Rise of America's Hospital System*. New York: Basic Books, 1987.

——. "Inward Vision and Outward Glance: The Shaping of the American Hospital, 1880–1914." In *Social History and Social Policy*, edited by David Rothman and Stanton Wheeler, 19–56. New York: Academic Press, 1981.

——. *No Other Gods: On Science and American Social Thought*. Baltimore: Johns Hopkins University Press, 1976.

——. "The Therapeutic Revolution: Medicine, Meaning, and Social Change in Nineteenth Century America." In *The Therapeutic Revolution: Essays in the Social History of American Medicine*, edited by Charles Rosenberg and Morris Vogel, 3–25. Philadelphia: University of Pennsylvania Press, 1979.

Rosenberg, Charles, and Morris Vogel, eds. *The Therapeutic Revolution: Essays in the Social History of American Medicine*. Philadelphia: University of Pennsylvania Press, 1979.

Rosenkrantz, Barbara. "Cart before Horse: Theory, Practice, and Professional Image in American Public Health, 1870–1920." *Bulletin of the History of Medicine and Allied Sciences* 29, no. 1 (1974): 55–73.

Rothenberg, Winifred. "The Emergence of Farm Labor Markets and the Transformation of the Rural Economy: Massachusetts, 1750–1855." *Journal of Economic History* 48 (1988): 537–66.

Rothman, Sheila. *Living in the Shadow of Death: Tuberculosis and the Social Experience of Illness in American History.* New York: Basic Books, 1994.

———. *Woman's Proper Place: A History of Changing Ideals and Practices, 1870 to the Present.* New York: Basic Books, 1978.

———. "Women's Clinics or Doctors' Offices: The Sheppard-Towner Act and the Promotion of Preventive Health Care." In *Social History and Social Policy*, edited by David Rothman and Stanton Wheeler, 175–202. New York: Academic Press, 1981.

Rothstein, William. *American Medical Schools and the Practice of Medicine: A History.* New York: Oxford University Press, 1987.

———. *American Physicians in the Nineteenth Century: From Seeds to Science.* Baltimore: Johns Hopkins University Press, 1972.

Rushing, Beth. "Market Explanations for Occupational Power: The Decline of Midwifery in Canada." *American Review of Canadian Studies* 21, no. 1 (1991): 7–27.

Salstrom, Paul. "Newer Appalachia as One of America's Last Frontiers." In *Appalachia in the Making: The Mountain South in the Nineteenth Century*, edited by Mary Beth Pudup, Dwight Billings, and Altina Waller. Chapel Hill: University of North Carolina Press, 1995.

Savage, Lon. *Thunder in the Mountains: The West Virginia Mine War, 1920–21.* South Charleston, W.Va.: Jalamap Publications, 1984.

Scott, Anne Firor. "After Suffrage: Southern Women in the Twenties." *Journal of Southern History* 30, no. 3 (August 1964): 298–318.

———. *Natural Allies: Women's Associations in American History.* Champaign: University of Illinois Press, 1993.

Scott, James. *Domination and the Arts of Resistance: Hidden Transcripts.* New Haven: Yale University Press, 1990.

———. *The Moral Economy of the Peasant: Rebellion and Subsistence in Southeast Asia.* New Haven: Yale University Press, 1976.

———. *Political Ideology in Malaysia: Reality and the Beliefs of an Elite.* New Haven: Yale University Press, 1968.

———. *Weapons of the Weak: Everyday Forms of Peasant Resistance.* New Haven: Yale University Press, 1985.

Scott, Shaunna. "Grannies, Mothers, and Babies: An Examination of Traditional Southern Appalachian Midwifery." *Central Issues in Anthropology* 4, no. 2 (1982): 17–30.

———. *Two Sides to Everything: The Construction of Class Consciousness in Harlan, Kentucky.* Albany: State University of New York Press, 1995.

Shackelford, Laurel, and Bill Weinberg, eds. *Our Appalachia: An Oral History.* Lexington: University Press of Kentucky, 1977.

Shapiro, Henry D. *Appalachia on Our Mind: The Southern Mountains and Mountaineers in the American Consciousness, 1870–1920.* Chapel Hill: University of North Carolina Press, 1978.

Sharp, Sharon. "Folk Medicine Practices: Women as Keepers and Carriers of Knowledge." *Women's Studies International Forum* 9, no. 3 (1986): 241–48.

Shaw, Stephanie J. "Black Club Women and the Creation of the National Association of Colored Women." *Journal of Women's History* 3, no. 2 (1991): 10–25.

Shelley, Karen, and Raymond Evans. "Women Folk Healers of Appalachia." In *Appalachia/America*, edited by Wilson Somerville, 209–17. Johnson City, Tenn.: Appalachian Consortium Press, 1981.

Shifflet, Crandall. *Coal Towns: Life, Work, and Culture of Company Towns in Southern Appalachia, 1880–1960.* Knoxville: University of Tennessee Press, 1991.

Shryock, Richard. *Medicine and Society in America: Historical Essays.* Baltimore: Johns Hopkins University Press, 1966.

Sklar, Kathryn Kish. "A Call for Comparisons." *American Historical Review* 95, no. 4 (1990): 1109–14.

———. "The Historical Foundations of Women's Power in the Creation of the American Welfare State, 1830–1930." In *Mothers of a New World: Maternalist Politics and the Origins of Welfare States*, edited by Seth Koven and Sonya Michel, 43–93. New York: Routledge, 1993.

———. "Hull House in the 1890s: A Community of Women Reformers." *Signs* 10, no. 4 (Summer 1985): 658–77.

———. "Hull House Maps and Papers: Social Science as Women's Work in the 1890s." In *The Social Survey in Historical Perspective, 1880–1940*, edited by Martin Bulmer, Kevin Bales, and Kathryn Kish Sklar, 111–47. New York: Cambridge University Press, 1991.

Skocpol, Theda. *Protecting Soldiers and Mothers: The Political Origins of Social Policy in the United States.* Cambridge: Belknap Press, 1992.

Skocpol, Theda, Marjorie Abend-Wein, Christopher Howard, and Susan Goodrich Lehmann. "Women's Associations and the Enactment of Mothers' Pension in the United States." *American Political Science Review* 87, no. 3 (1987): 686–701.

Smith, Barbara Ellen. *Digging Our Own Graves: Coal Miners and the Struggle over Black Lung Disease.* Philadelphia: Temple University Press, 1987.

———. "Walk-ons in the Third Act: The Role of Women in Appalachian Historiography." *Journal of Appalachian Studies* 4, no. 1 (Spring 1998): 5–28.

———. *Women of the Rural South: Economic Status and Prospects.* Lexington, Ky.: Southeast Women's Employment Coalition, 1986.

———, ed. *Neither Separate Nor Equal: Women, Race, and Class in the U.S. South.* Philadelphia: Temple University Press, 1999.

Stage, Sarah. *Female Complaints: Lydia Pinkham and the Business of Women's Medicine.* New York: Norton, 1979.

Starr, Paul. *The Social Transformation of American Medicine: The Rise of a Sovereign Profession and the Making of a Vast Empire.* New York: Basic Books, 1982.

Stevens, Rosemary. *American Medicine and the Public Interest*. New Haven: Yale University Press, 1971.

Susie, Deborah Ann. *In the Ways of Our Grandmothers: A Cultural View of Twentieth Century Midwifery in Florida*. Athens: University of Georgia Press, 1988.

Tams, W. P., Jr. *The Smokeless Coal Fields of West Virginia: A Brief History*. Parsons, W.Va.: McClain, 1963.

Taylor, Lloyd, Jr. *The Medical Profession and Social Reform, 1885–1945*. New York: St. Martin's, 1974.

Thurmond, Walter R. *The Logan Coal Field of West Virginia*. Parsons, W.Va.: McClain, 1964.

Tice, Karen. "School-Work and Mother-Work: The Interplay of Maternalism and Cultural Politics in the Educational Narratives of Kentucky Settlement Workers, 1910–1930." *Journal of Appalachian Studies* 4, no. 2 (Fall 1998): 191–224.

Tiffin, Susan. *In Whose Best Interest?: Child Welfare Reform in the Progressive Era*. Westport, Conn.: Greenwood Press, 1982.

Toynbee, Arnold. *A Study of History*. Vol. 2. New York: Oxford University Press, 1947.

Trattner, Walter, ed. *Social Welfare or Social Control?: Some Historical Reflections on Regulating the Poor*. Knoxville: University of Tennessee Press, 1983.

Trolander, Judith. *Professionalism and Social Change: From the Settlement House to Neighborhood Centers, 1886 to the Present*. New York: Columbia University Press, 1987.

Trotter, Joe. *Coal, Class, and Color: Blacks in Southern West Virginia, 1915–1932*. Urbana: University of Illinois, 1990.

Turner, Carolyn Clay, and Carolyn Hay Traum. *John C. C. Mayo: Cumberland Capitalist*. Pikeville, Ky.: Pikeville College Press, 1983.

Walkowitz, Daniel. "The Making of a Feminine Professional Identity." *American Historical Review* 95, no. 4 (October 1990): 1051–75.

Waller, Altina L. *Feud: Hatfields, McCoys, and Social Change in Appalachia, 1860–1900*. Chapel Hill: University of North Carolina Press, 1988.

Walsh, Mary Roth. *Doctors Wanted—No Women Need Apply: Sexual Barriers in the Medical Profession, 1835–1975*. New Haven: Yale University Press, 1977.

Ware, Susan. *Beyond Suffrage: Women in the New Deal*. Cambridge: Harvard University Press, 1981.

Warner, John Harley. "Ideals of Science and Their Discontents in Late Nineteenth-Century American Medicine." *Isis* 82, no. 313 (September 1991): 454–78.

———. *The Therapeutic Perspective: Medical Practice, Knowledge, and Identity in America, 1820–1885*. Cambridge: Harvard University Press, 1986.

Warren, Harlow. *Beckley, USA*. Beckley, W.Va.: Privately published, 1955.

Weber, Max. *On Charisma and Institution Building*. Edited by S. N. Eisenstadt. Chicago: University of Chicago Press, 1968.

Weiner, Deborah. "Middlemen of the Coalfields: The Role of Jews in the Economy of Southern West Virginia Coal Towns, 1890–1950." *Journal of Appalachian Studies* 4, no. 1 (Spring 1998): 29–56.

Weller, Jack. *Yesterday's People: Life in Contemporary Appalachia*. Lexington: University Press of Kentucky, 1965.

Wells, Mildred White. *Unity in Diversity: The History of the General Federation of Women's Clubs*. Washington, D.C.: General Federation of Women's Clubs, 1953.

Wertz, Richard, and Dorothy Wertz. *Lying-in: A History of Childbirth in America*. New York: Free Press, 1977.

Whisnant, David. *All That Is Native and Fine: The Politics of Culture in an American Region*. Chapel Hill: University of North Carolina Press, 1983.

———. *Modernizing the Mountaineer: People, Power, and Planning in Appalachia*. New York: Burt Franklin, 1980.

Whites, Lee Ann. "The De Graffenreid Controversy: Class, Race, and Gender in the New South." *Journal of Southern History* 54, no. 3 (August 1988): 449–78.

Wiebe, Robert H. *The Search for Order, 1877–1920*. New York: Hill and Wang, 1967.

Wilding, Paul. *Professional Power and Social Welfare*. London: Routledge and Kegan Paul, 1982.

INDEX

French-Eversole feud, 23
Friedson, Eliot, 7, 8, 42, 48
Frontier Nursing Service, 11, 88,
    95–97, 103, 126; and attempts
    to displace lay healers, 116–17;
    cooperation with medical estab-
    lishment, 115; as example of
    female-directed organization, 113;
    physicians' tolerance for, 136–37
Fry, Francis, Dr., 20
Furman, Lucy, 10, 26, 92

Gaventa, John, 3
General Federation of Women's
    Clubs (GFWC), 9, 73, 74, 84,
    103, 110
"Good mothers," 9–10
Gore, Howard, 59
Graduate Nurses' Association of Vir-
    ginia, 142
Graham, John T., Dr., 38

Haines, Blanche, Dr., 138
Hall, Eula, 156
Haller, I. G., Dr., 21, 23
Harlan County, Kentucky, 17–18
Harvard University, 43, 47
Harvey, Vera, 126
Hatfield, "Devil Anse," 31, 37
Hatfield, Henry, Dr., 31, 36, 39
Hatfield, S. D., Dr., 37
Hatton, Benjamin, Dr., 22
Hazard, Kentucky, 91
Hennen, John, 13
Heroic medicine, 5, 16, 24–25, 26
Hewitt, Nancy, 73
Hindman Settlement School, 11,
    90–93, 97, 98, 125, 126
Hoffert, Sylvia, 7
Homeopathic Hospital College of
    Ohio, 22
Homeopaths, 8
Hospital College of Medicine, 21, 45
Hospitals constructed by physicians,
    38–39, 83
Hull House, 89, 96

Hume, H. H., Dr., 53, 81
Hume, Hundly Gazelle, 80

Infant and maternal mortality,
    123–24
Inscoe, John, 3
Internships completed by Appala-
    chian doctors, 46–48
Ireland, W. Bertram, 105
Island Creek Coal Company, 133

Jackson County, Kentucky, 55
Jane Todd Crawford Fund, 149
Jefferson Medical College, 21, 22,
    23, 48
John George Hohman's Pow-Wows, 26
Johns Hopkins University, 43, 47
Jones, Harriet, Dr., 82, 112
Joynes, Levin, 21

Kaufman, Maurice, Dr., 52
Kentucky Board of Health, 95
Kentucky Bureau of Maternal and
    Child Health, 68, 137
Kentucky Committee for Mothers
    and Babies, 96
Kentucky Federation of Women's
    Clubs, 74, 75, 85, 91, 93, 95
Kentucky School of Medicine, 22,
    44
Kentucky Society for the Prevention
    of Blindness, 95
Kentucky State Medical Society, 50,
    51, 58, 115, 119, 133, 149, 173
    (n. 85); opposition to UMWA
    Welfare and Retirement Fund,
    154
Kentucky University Medical
    Department, 45
Kerns, W. W., Dr., 128
Kincaid, J. D., Dr., 21, 23, 56
Knott County Medical Association,
    52
Koch, Robert, 24
Koven, Seth, 102, 152

Mingo County, West Virginia, 30, 144

Mingo County Medical Society, 53, 61

Monongalia County, West Virginia, 128–30

Monongalia County Medical Society, 140; opposition to county public health unit, 128–30

Morgantown, West Virginia, 130

Moser, Joan, 26

Mountain Fund for Needy Eye Sufferers, 95, 97, 132

Mud Creek Clinic, 155–56

Muncy, Robin, 10, 11, 89

Municipal housekeeping, 10, 72

Murdock, H. S., 93

National Baby Week, 86

National Health Service Corps, 157

National Organization of Public Health Nurses, 111

Neel, H. F., Dr., 32

Neville, Linda, 88, 93–97, 132; crusade against lay midwifery, 119–20, 135–36

Noe, Kenneth, 3

Norfolk and Western Railroad, 30, 39, 78

Numbers, Ronald, 127

Office of Economic Opportunity, 155

Old Dominion Hospital, 44

Osteopaths, 54, 59

Painter, Tim, Dr., 24

Park, J. S., Dr., 21

Pasteur, Louis, 24

Patent medicines, 27

Perry County, Kentucky, 17, 23, 91

Pettit, Katherine, 10, 90, 92–94, 96

Physicians: alliance with clubwomen against lay midwifery, 119–20, 135–36; alliance with

state government to promote medical advances, 54–56; campaigns against sectarians, 41; as charitable agents, 110–11; claims to scientific knowledge, 7; and coal operators, 29; distrust of growing independence of public health nurses, 138–42; diversity of medical training during industrialization, 34–36; expectation of payment in cash, 32–33; generational conflicts among, 54–57; graduation from elite institutions, 47–48; movement into preventive care, 123, 127; nativity of, 48; new markets for, 6, 106; non-degreed physicians, 22–23; objections to public health units, 107–8, 128–31; opposition to licensing of lay midwives in West Virginia in 1990s, 158–59; opposition to Sheppard-Towner Act and training of lay midwives, 134–36; opposition to UMWA Welfare and Retirement Fund and Miners' Memorial Hospital Fund, 154–55; postgraduate training, 48; in preindustrial Appalachia, 17–18, 21–24; promotion of proprietary medical model, 124–26, 132–34; recent arrivals in Appalachia, 6, 33–34, 48; rejection of privately funded public health campaigns, 131–34; scarcity of obstetricians in West Virginia in 1990s, 157; struggle for professional recognition, 69–70

Piedmont Sanitorium, 142

Pike County, Kentucky, 31, 32

Pine Mountain Settlement School, 11, 90, 92, 97, 117, 126

Polk's Medical Register, 33, 35, 43

Preceptors, 20, 22

Price, Lucille, 80, 112

Price, Samuel, Dr., 80

Price, William, Dr., 37

Thompson, Penelope, 64–65
Tice, Karen, 2, 11, 90
Trachoma, 93, 116, 118
Transylvania University, 22, 24
Tug River valley, 25, 30

United Mine Workers of America
    (UMWA), 144, 153–54
United Mine Workers' Welfare and
    Retirement Fund, 154, 155
University College of Medicine, 46,
    53
University of Liverpool, 21
University of Louisville, 5, 16, 20,
    21, 31, 36, 37–38, 43–47, 55, 56
University of Maryland, 22
University of Michigan, 43
University of Pennsylvania, 21, 43,
    47
University of Tennessee Medical
    School, 30
University of Virginia, 22, 37, 39,
    48, 53
U.S. Coal and Oil Company, 31
U.S. Coal Commission, 104–5
U.S. Public Health Service, 139

Veech, Annie, Dr., 68, 137
Virginia Board of Health, 131
Virginia Bureau of Public Health
    Nursing, 137
Virginia Federation of Women's
    Clubs, 75, 76, 85, 107, 143
Virginia Medical Monthly, 54
Virginia State Board of Medicine, 58
Virginia State Medical Examining
    Board, 57

Waldron, M. H., Dr., 66
Waller, Altina, 3, 31
Warner, John Harley, 3–4, 24–25
Weather Vane, 141
West Virginia Anti-Tuberculosis
    League, 81
West Virginia Board of Health, 86
West Virginia Coal and Coke, 87

West Virginia Department of Health,
    139
West Virginia Division of Child
    Hygiene and Public Health Nurs-
    ing, 112, 138, 140
West Virginia Federation of Wom-
    en's Clubs, 1, 75, 79, 81, 82, 110,
    126, 140, 144, 145; Department
    of Public Health, 143; Public
    Health Committee, 80, 85, 107
West Virginia Medical Journal, 52
West Virginia Nursing Licensure
    Board, 141–42
West Virginia Public Health Associa-
    tion, 150
West Virginia State Medical Associa-
    tion, 36, 43, 46–47, 48, 50, 54,
    60, 77, 85, 127, 133, 136, 141, 158
West Virginia State Nurses' Associa-
    tion, 81, 140, 141
West Virginia State Women's Coun-
    cil, 147
Wheeler, C. W., Dr., 22
Whisnant, David, 91, 97, 98
White, Isabel, 64–65
White, Susan, 63–65
Williamson, West Virginia, 29, 143
Women's auxiliaries, 12, 145–50;
    deference to medical societies,
    147; influence on independent
    women's clubs, 148–49; as
    replacements for independent
    women's clubs, 150–51
Women's Auxiliary of the Kentucky
    State Medical Society, 146–47,
    149
Women's Auxiliary of the Letcher
    County, Kentucky, Medical Soci-
    ety, 149
Women's Auxiliary of the Medical
    Society of Virginia, 146–47
Women's Auxiliary of the West Vir-
    ginia State Medical Association,
    146–48, 150
Women's Christian Temperance
    Union, 91, 92, 145

Women's Club of Omar, West Virginia, 87–88

Woodson, William, Dr., 142

World War I: and women's health promotions, 83–84

Wythe County Medical Society, 52

Wytheville, Virginia, 22, 24, 38

Zeigler, Frances Helen, 142

Index